Recent Developments in Myelodysplastic Syndromes

Edited by Ota Fuchs

Published in London, United Kingdom

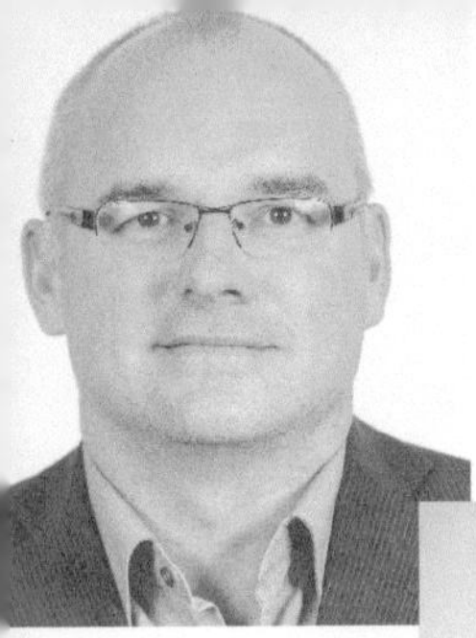
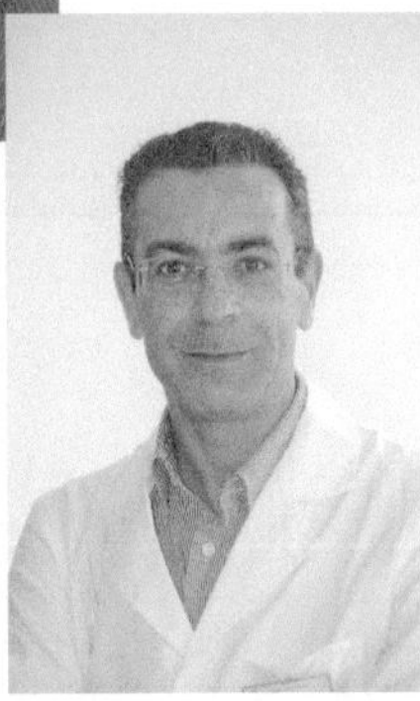
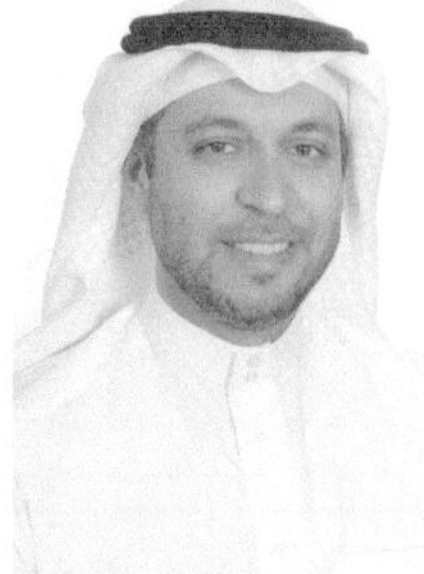
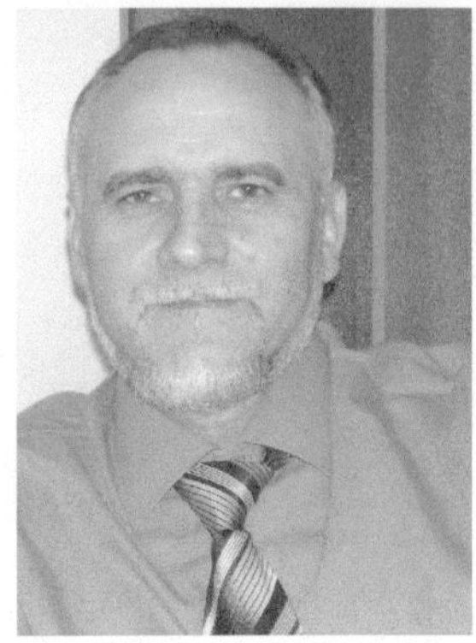
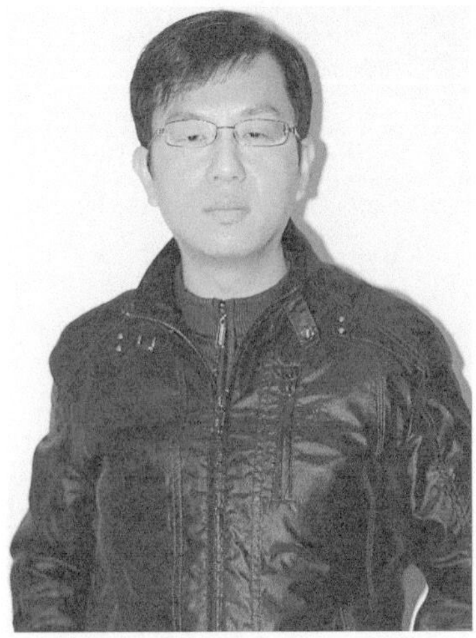
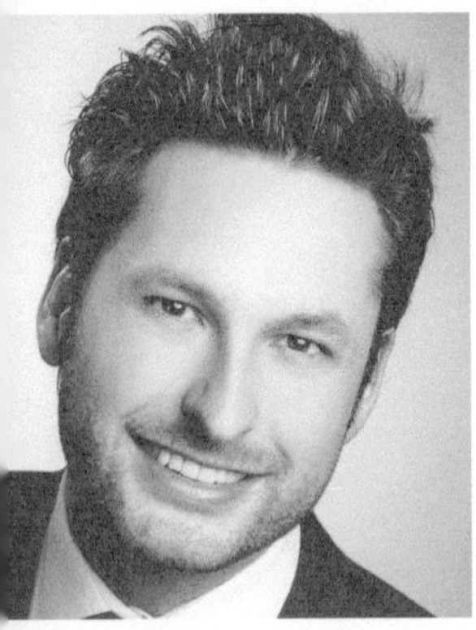
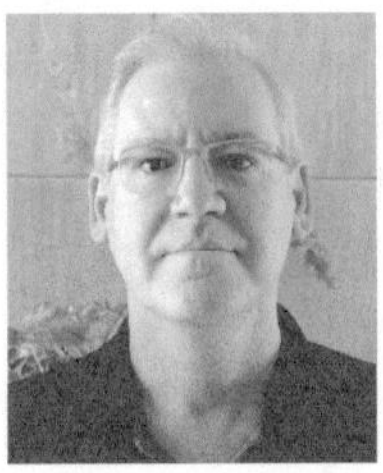

IntechOpen

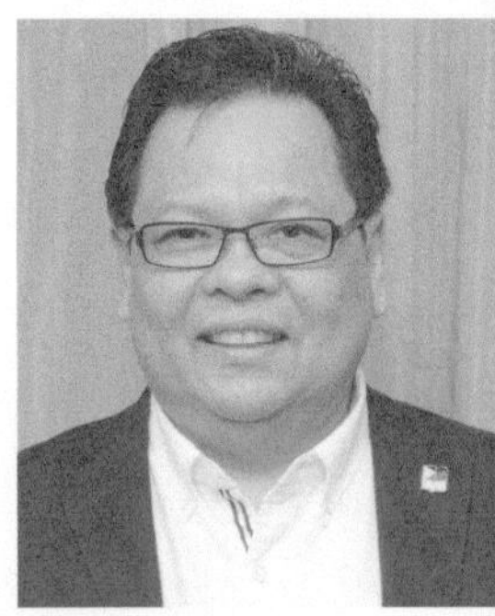
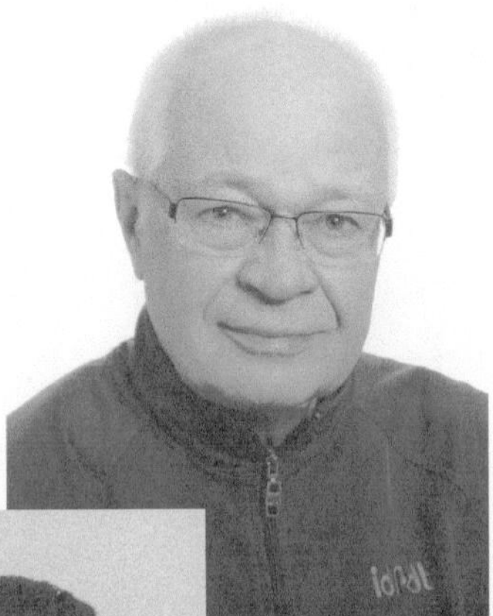
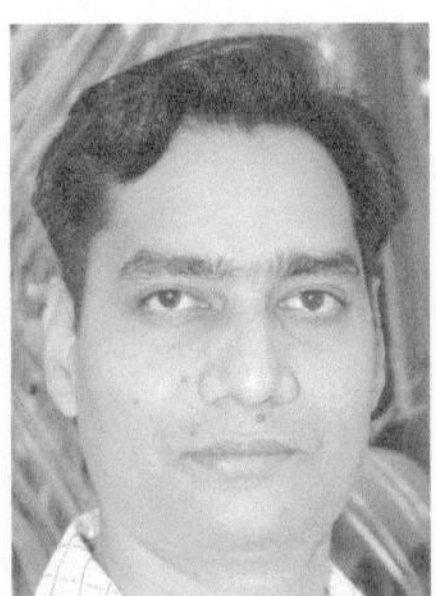
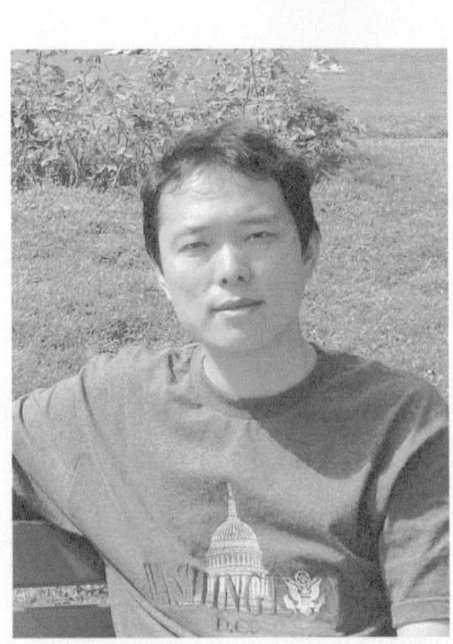
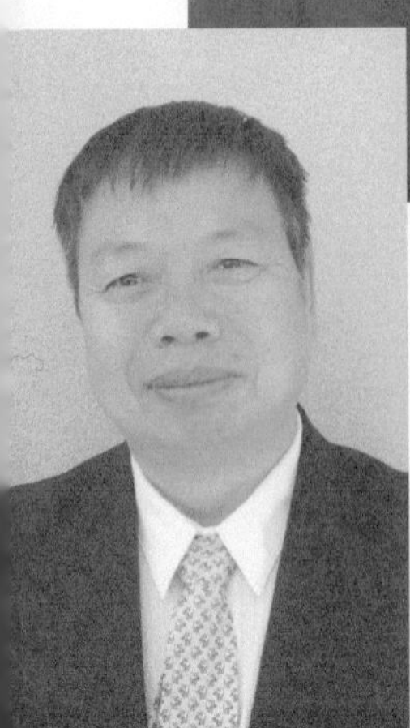
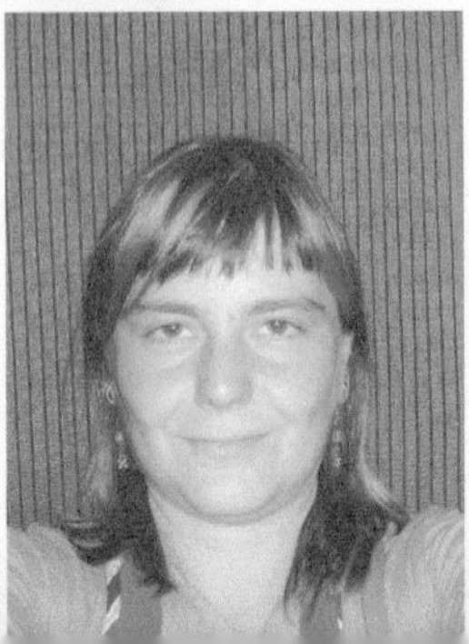

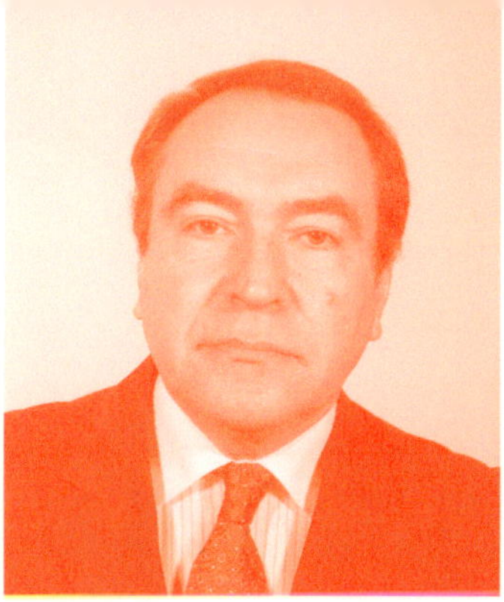

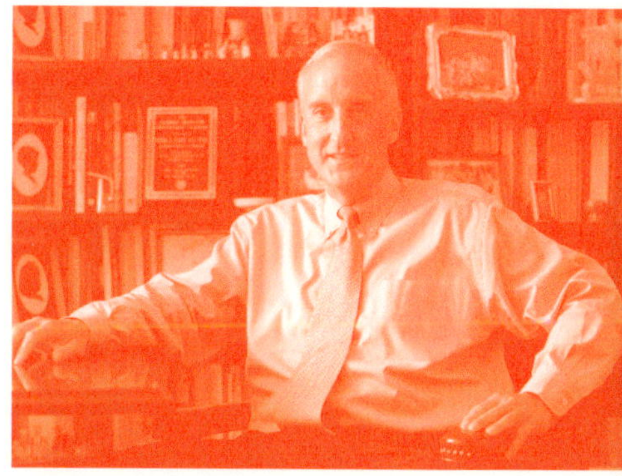

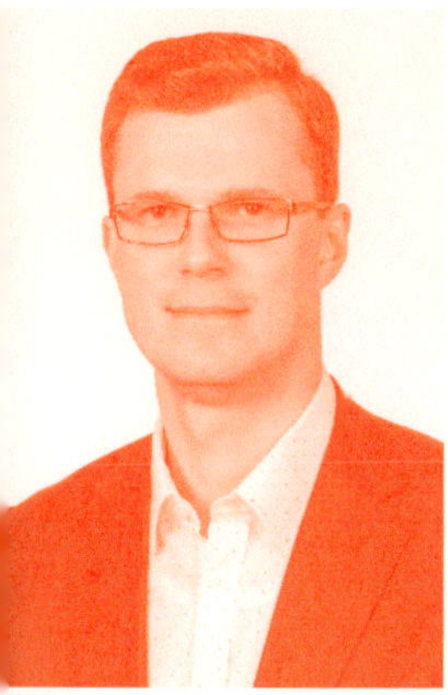

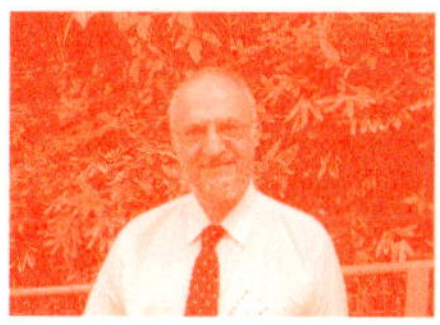

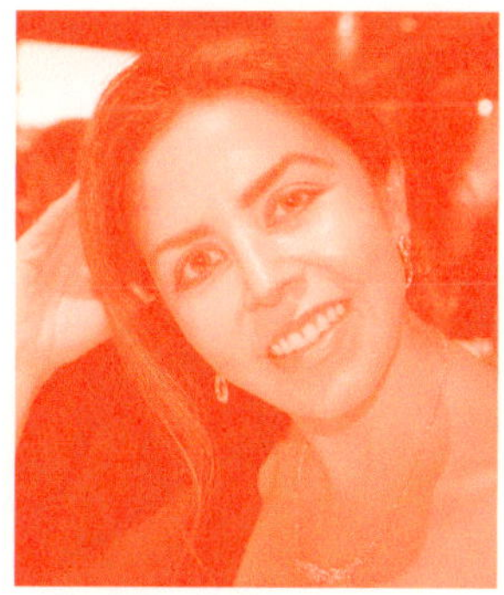

Supporting open minds since 2005

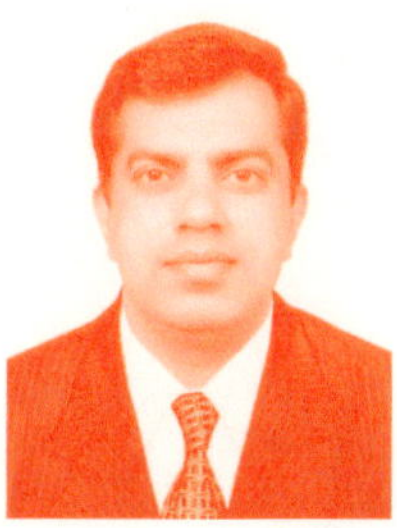

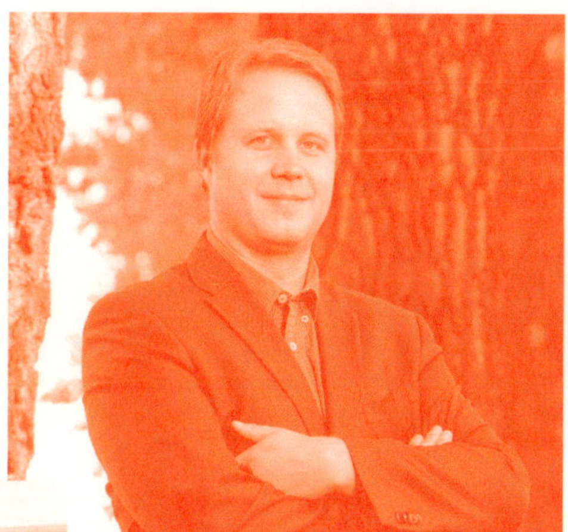

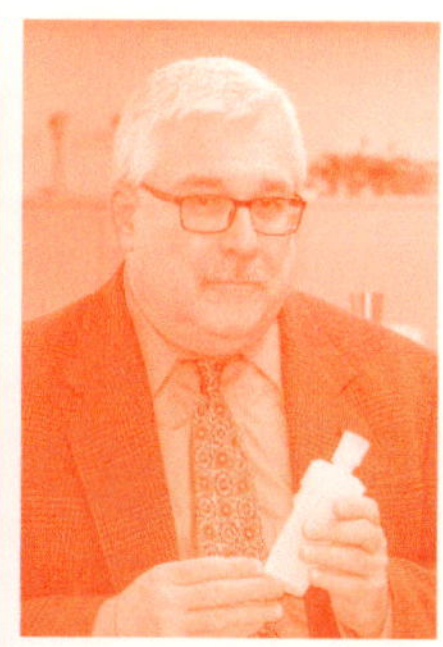

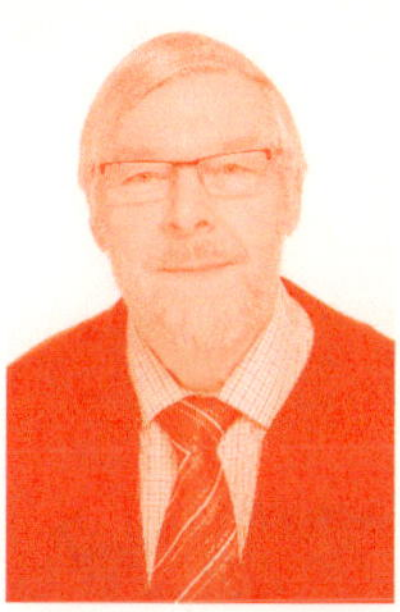

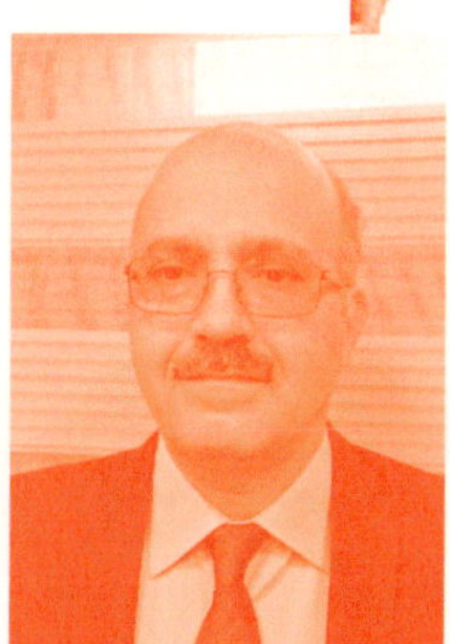

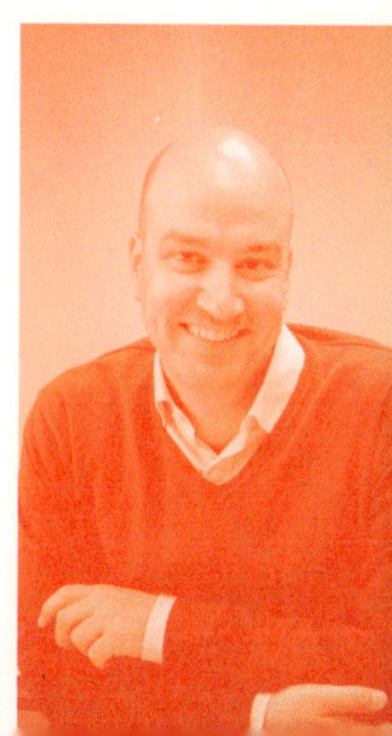

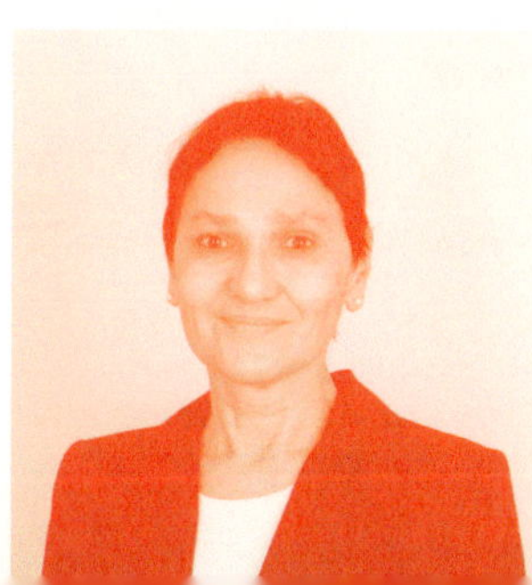

Recent Developments in Myelodysplastic Syndromes
http://dx.doi.org/10.5772/intechopen.73936
Edited by Ota Fuchs

Contributors
Michaela Dost√°lov√° Merkerov√°, Andrea Hru≈°tincov√°, Katarina Szikszai, Zdenƒõk Krejƒç√≠k, Nikoleta Loudov√°, Kam A. Newman, Mojtaba Akhtari, Sheda Heidarian, Selma D\'Silva, Meenakshi Singh, Sunil Rajadhyaksha, Gamal Abdul Hamid, Safa Shukry, Abdulwahab Al-Nehmi, Wanxing Chai-Ho, Gary Schiller, Ota Fuchs

First published in London, United Kingdom, 2019 by IntechOpen
IntechOpen is the global imprint of INTECHOPEN LIMITED, registered in England and Wales, registration number: 11086078, The Shard, 25th floor, 32 London Bridge Street
London, SE19SG - United Kingdom
Printed in Croatia

British Library Cataloguing-in-Publication Data
A catalogue record for this book is available from the British Library

Additional hard copies can be obtained from orders@intechopen.com

Recent Developments in Myelodysplastic Syndromes
Edited by Ota Fuchs
p. cm.
Print ISBN 978-1-78985-477-0
Online ISBN 978-1-78985-478-7

For EU product safety concerns:
IN TECH d.o.o., Prolaz Marije Krucifikse Kozulić 3, 51000 Rijeka, Croatia, info@intechopen.com or visit our website at intechopen.com.

Meet the editor

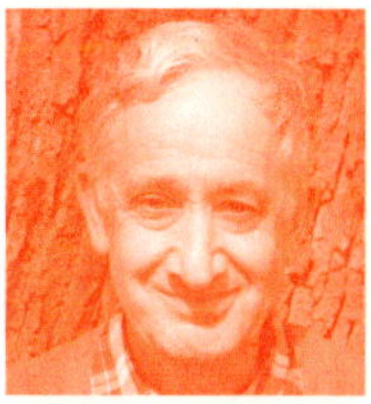

Ota Fuchs graduated from the Chemical Technological University, Prague, Czech Republic, in 1971. He obtained his PhD in Biochemistry from the Faculty of Natural Sciences, Charles University, Prague, in 1981. He is employed as a senior scientist at the Institute of Hematology and Blood Transfusion, Prague. He undertook a visiting scientist short-term affiliation in the Beatson Institute for Cancer Research, Glasgow, UK, the Institute of Experimental Medicine of the Russian Academy of Medical Sciences in St. Petersburg, Russia, and in the Lady Davis Institute for Medical Research, Jewish General Hospital, Montreal, Canada. He was the principal investigator of five projects for the Internal Grant Agency of the Ministry of Health of the Czech Republic and of one grant project for the Grant Agency of the Czech Republic. He is a member of the Czech Medical Society J.E. Purkyne and the Czech MDS Group.

Contents

Preface

Genome and exome sequencing together with targeted deep-sequencing studies have defined several gene mutations in almost every myelodysplastic syndrome (MDS) patient. These mutations can impact disease phenotype, prognosis and disease progression. However, there are many non-pathogenic mutations, and most mutations are not specific for MDS. Applying this information clinically is in progress even if the clinical impact of some mutations remains controversial. Several mutations will likely be incorporated into future prognostic scoring systems. Great progress has also been reached in the studies of non-coding RNAs in MDS. It is possible that they will be used in MDS diagnostics and prognosis. Big advancements in the studies of immune mechanisms in MDS have been achieved and translated into clinical studies of immunotherapies in MDS. Innate and adaptive immune pathways are excessively active in the niche of hematopoietic cells in MDS. Common etiological mechanisms of MDS and autoimmune diseases is possible because these diseases are often associated with MDS. Unfortunately, no new drugs have been approved for MDS since approval by the Food and Drug Administration of azacitidine in 2004, lenalidomide in 2005, and decitabine in 2006. The European Medicines Agency approved azacitidine in 2008 and lenalidomide in 2013. This progress in many aspects of MDS warrants this new book about this heterogeneous group of clonal neoplasms arising from hematopoietic stem cells, and characterized by inefficient hematopoiesis, peripheral cytopenias, frequent karyotypic abnormalities, risk of clonal evolution, and transformation to acute myeloid leukemia, three years after the last book about MDS published by IntechOpen.

This book provides a review of several fields of MDS not only for research workers and clinicians, but also for medical students with an interest in MDS. The first introductory chapter deals with recent progress in this area. The second chapter provides a review of diagnosis and classification of MDS. Chapter 3 discusses the association of MDS and autoimmune disorders. Chapter 4 introduces immune dysregulation in MDS. The fifth chapter analyzes an update on pathophysiology and management of MDS. The last chapter discusses non-coding RNAs in MDS.

Ota Fuchs, PhD
Institute of Hematology and Blood Transfusion,
Department of Genomics,
Prague, Czech Republic

Chapter 1

Introductory Chapter: Progress in Myelodysplastic Syndrome Area

Ota Fuchs

1. Advances in our knowledge of cytogenetic abnormalities and gene mutations

Myelodysplastic syndromes (MDS) constitute a group of age-associated heterogeneous clonal hematopoietic disorders characterized by ineffective hematopoiesis with peripheral cytopenias, dysplasia, and an increased risk of progression to acute myeloid leukemia (AML) [1–6]. About 50% of cases of MDS are characterized by the presence of cytogenetic abnormalities. Losses of chromosomal material as del(5q), del(20q), monosomy 7 or del(7q), and del(Y) are most common cytogenetic abnormalities and are more frequent than gains of chromosomal material as trisomy 8 or trisomy 21 [7].

MDS are caused by abnormalities in many genes. The great progress in analysis of these mutations and in elucidation of relationships between gene mutations and clinical phenotypes of these disorders was achieved. Somatic mutations were found in more than 90%. Next-generation sequencing (NGS) detected about 10 different mutations in almost every patient with MDS. The majority of these mutations are nonpathogenic passenger mutations. However, one or more driver mutations in most patients with MDS are associated with the pathogenesis of MDS. Gene mutations affect proteins involved in various important cell processes as RNA-splicing, DNA methylation, histone and chromatin modifications, signal transduction, transcription (transcription factors), tumor suppressor (*TP53*), *RAS* pathway, and separation of sister chromatids during cell division (cohesion complex) [4, 8–10].

RNA-splicing and DNA methylation mutations occur early and are known as founding mutations. Other mutations are called subclonal mutations. No MDS-specific mutations exist. Strongly represented mutations in genes coding for proteins involved in DNA methylation, such as *TET2*, *DNMT3A*, and *ASXL1*, are common also in older individuals with normal blood count (clonal hematopoiesis of indeterminate potential/CHIP/) [11, 12]. Until now, mutations in *TP53*, *EZH2*, *RUNX1*, and *SF3B1* predict independently overall survival (OS) of MDS patients. The first three mutations are associated with shorter OS but the last mutation is connected with better survival in refractory anemia with ring sideroblast (MDS-RS) and with thrombocytosis (RARS-T) [13, 14]. *SF3B1* mutations are present in about 80% of MDS-RS and correlates with its development. *SF3B1* mutations could alter the expression of the gene for ABCB7 transporter and abnormally regulate iron homeostasis in mitochondria mediating the phenotype of acquired MDS-RS [15]. Effects of other mutations are not clear up to now and results are often controversial.

We lack clinical methods to stop clonal development from relatively benign state of CHIP to malignancy. Especially, *TP53*-mutant clones induce progress to therapy-related MDS/AML. Therapy-related myeloid neoplasms have mutations in *TP53* and epigenetic modifying genes, instead of mutations in tyrosine kinase and spliceosome genes [16]. The possible treatments are now the use of hypomethylating agents or in future anti-inflammatory therapy and clonally selective immunotherapies.

MDS are associated with genomic instability and extensive DNA damage caused by deficient repair mechanisms. Aberrations in DNA damage response/repair genes other than *TP53* and some genes involved in DNA damage checkpoints are rare. Differential expression of homologous recombination DNA repair-associated genes during MDS progression was detected and could be confirmed as new biomarkers related to pathogenesis and poor prognosis in MDS [17, 18].

2. Advance in our understanding of del(5q) myelodysplastic syndrome pathogenesis and its treatment with lenalidomide

The greatest progress was achieved in the study of molecular pathogenesis of del(5q) MDS disease phenotype and its treatment by immunomodulatory or cereblon-binding drug lenalidomide [2, 19–35]. Ebert et al. described that impaired ribosome biosynthesis due to *RPS14* (ribosomal protein 14 of the small ribosome subunit) gene haploinsufficiency leads to the E3 ubiquitin ligase HDM2 (human homolog to mouse double minute 2, major negative regulator of p53) inactivation by free ribosomal proteins, particularly RPL11 [36]. HDM2 degradation drives p53-mediated apoptosis of erythroid cells carrying the del(5q) aberration. This p53-mediated apoptosis of erythroid cells is a key effector of hypoplastic anemia in MDS patients with del(5q) [36]. *RPS14* haploinsufficiency causes a block in erythroid differentiation mediated by calprotectin (the heterodimeric S100 calcium-binding proteins S100A8 and S100A9) [37]. Proinflammatory proteins, S100A9 and tumor necrosis factor-α, suppress the effect of erythropoietin in MDS [38]. Some patients originally considered as MDS patients without del(5q) can have a phenotype of atypical 5q− syndrome and can be sensitive to lenalidomide therapy because they have diminutive somatic deletions in the 5q region. These deletions were not identified by fluorescence in situ hybridization or cytogenetic testing but by single nucleotide polymorphism array genotyping [39]. Low RPS14 expression in 50–70% MDS patients without del(5q) confers higher apoptosis rate of nucleated erythrocytes and predicts prolonged survival [40, 41].

What is the mechanism of lenalidomide in del(5q) MDS based on what has been achieved and elucidated to date? Lenalidomide stabilizes E3 ubiquitin ligase HDM2, thereby accelerating p53 degradation [42, 43]. Lenalidomide inhibits phosphatases PP2a and Cdc25c (coregulators of cell cycle which genes are very commonly deleted in del(5q) MDS) with consequent G2 arrest of del(5q) MDS progenitors and their apoptosis. PP2a and Cdc25c inhibition by lenalidomide suppress HDM2 autoubiquitination and subsequent degradation. Thus, lenalidomide has been shown to not only reverse apoptosis within the erythroid compartment, but also directly induce apoptosis of the myeloid clone in del(5q) MDS [44, 45]. Lenalidomide upregulates expression of other two haploinsufficient genes located on chromosome 5q, genes for microRNAs (miR-145 and miR-146a) [46]. These miRs are involved in Toll-like receptor pathway, IL-6 induction, and regulation of megakaryopoiesis [20].

Ito et al. discovered that thalidomide (founding member of immunomodulatory drugs/IMiDs/) binds cereblon (CRBN) in the terminal C-region (parts of exons 10 and 11 of the *CRBN* gene code this IMiD binding region) [47]. Several researchers confirmed CRBN as target of lenalidomide in multiple myeloma (MM), lymphoma, chronic lymphocytic leukemia, and del(5q) MDS [48]. CRBN is the ubiquitously expressed 51 kDa protein with a putative role in cerebral development, especially memory and learning [49, 50].

Our group found that del(5q) MDS patients (the so-called 5q minus syndrome) have higher levels of full-length CRBN mRNA than other patients with lower risk MDS, linking higher levels of a known lenalidomide target CRBN and del(5q) MDS subgroup known to be especially sensitive to lenalidomide [51].

CRBN is a member and substrate receptor of the cullin 4 RING E3 ubiquitin ligase complex (CRL4). CRBN recruits substrate proteins to the CRL4 complex for ubiquitination and the subsequent degradation in proteasomes. IMiDs binds to CRBN in CRL4 complex and block normal endogenous substrates (CRBN and the homeobox transcription factor MEIS2 in multiple myeloma/MM/) from binding to CRL4 for ubiquitination and degradation [52]. After IMID binding to CRBN, CRL4 complex is recruiting transcription factors Ikaros (IKZF1) and Aiolos (IKZF3) for ubiquitination and degradation in MM cells [53]. Degradation of these transcription factors explains lenalidomide's growth inhibition of MM cells and increased interleukin-2 (IL-2) release from T cells. However, it is unlikely that degradation of IKZF1 and IKZF3 accounts for lenalidomide's activity in MDS with del(5q). Fink et al. identified a novel target casein kinase1A1 (CSNK1A1) by quantitative proteomics in the myeloid cell line KG-1 [54]. CSNK1A1 is encoded in the del(5q) commonly deleted region and the gene is haploinsufficient. Lenalidomide treatment leads to increased ubiquitination of the remaining CSNK1A1 and decreased protein abundance. CSNK1A1 negatively regulates β-catenin which drives stem cell self-renewal, and *CSNK1A1* haploinsufficiency causes the initial clonal expansion in patients with the del(5q) MDS and contributes to the pathogenesis of del(5q) MDS. The further inhibition of CSNK1A1 in del(5q) MDS is associated with del(5q) failure and p53 activation. The inhibition of CSNK1A1 reduced RPS6 phosphorylation, induced p53 expression and growth inhibition, and triggered myeloid differentiation program. TP53-null leukemia did not respond to CSNK1A1 inhibition, strongly supporting the importance of the p53 expression for the yield of CSNK1A1 inhibition. *CSNK1A1* mutations have been recently found in 5–18% of MDS patients with del(5q) [55]. These mutations are associated similarly to the effect of *TP53* mutations with rise to a poor prognosis in del(5q) MDS [56]. Other studies did not find impact of *CSNK1A1* mutations on lenalidomide treatment in del(5q) MDS [57, 58].

Even if the treatment of del(5q) MDS patients with lenalidomide is very efficient, 50% of treated patients relapse after 2–3 years. Martinez-Hoyer et al. found that low platelet count and occurrence of additional mutations, mainly *TP53* mutations induce lenalidomide resistance [59–61]. They used whole genome sequencing and observed in several resistant patients mutations in *RUNX1* gene or decreased amount of *RUNX1* transcript without aberration in *TP53* [59]. Results were verified in model system of two human del(5q) lines, MDS-L and KG-1a. *RUNX1* knock-out or RUNX1 shRNA increased proliferation and reduced apoptosis in lenalidomide-treated cells with decreased *RUNX1* transcript. Therefore, effect of lenalidomide in del(5q) requires functional RUNX1. Similar results were obtained with *TP53* knock-out cells. Both *RUNX1* and *TP53* transcripts cooperate and alter the activity of GATA2 transcriptional complex [59].

3. Studies on lenalidomide use also in lower risk non-del(5q) MDS treatment and new possible therapies

While CSNK1A1 is $CRL4^{CRBN}$ target in del(5q) MDS, $CRL4^{CRBN}$ targets in lower risk non-del(5q) remain to be determined. The mechanism of action of lenalidomide is still unclear in non-del(5q) MDS cells. Recent evidence shows that lenalidomide directly improves erythropoietin receptor (EPOR) signaling by EPOR upregulation mediated by a posttranscriptional mechanism [62]. Lenalidomide stabilizes the EPOR protein by inhibition of the E3 ubiquitin ligase RNF41 (ring finger protein 41, also known as neuregulin receptor degradation protein-1/Nrdp1/ and fetal liver ring finger/FLRF/) responsible for EPOR polyubiquitination and next degradation [62] and induces lipid raft assembly to enhance EPOR signaling in MDS erythroid progenitors [63, 64].

After failure of ESAs, lenalidomide yields red blood cell transfusion independence in 20–30% of lower risk non-del(5q) MDS. Indeed, several observations suggest an additive effect of ESA and lenalidomide in this situation [65, 66] and also in del(5q) MDS patients [67]. Synthetic corticosteroids (dexamethasone and prednisone) are also able to potentiate the effect of lenalidomide or combination of lenalidomide and erythropoietin [67–69].

Basiorka et al. and Sallman et al. reported activation of the NLRP3 inflammasome in MDS [70, 71]. NRLP3 drives clonal expansion and pyroptotic cell death. Independent of genotype, MDS hematopoietic stem and progenitor cells (HSPCs) overexpress inflammasome proteins. Activated NLRP3 complexes direct then activation of caspase-1, generation of interleukin-1β (IL-1β) and IL-18, and pyroptotic cell death. Mechanistically, pyroptosis is triggered by the alarmin S100A9 that is found in excess in MDS HSPCs and bone marrow plasma. Further, like somatic gene mutations, S100A9-induced signaling activates NADPH oxidase (NOX) and increasing levels of reactive oxygen species (ROS). ROS initiate cation influx, cell swelling, and β-catenin activation. Knockdown of NLRP3 or caspase-1, neutralization of S100A9, and pharmacologic inhibition of NLRP3 or NOX suppress pyroptosis, ROS generation, and nuclear β-catenin in MDSs and are sufficient to restore effective hematopoiesis. Thus, alarmins and founder gene mutations in MDSs cause a common redox-sensitive inflammasome circuit. They are new candidates for therapeutic intervention.

Not only apoptosis and pyroptosis are involved in increased cell death in MDS. Recently, possible further mechanism of cell death, necroptosis, in MDS has been described [72, 73]. Necroptosis is like pyroptosis associated with membrane permeabilization and the release of damage-associated molecular patterns (DAMPs) such as alarmins. Alarmins bind Toll-like receptor 4 (TLR4) and activate the transcription factor NF-κB and inflammation [74].

The effects of lenalidomide in non-del(5q) are thought to be secondary to modulation of the immune system. Hyperactivated T cells inhibit hematopoiesis. Immunosuppressive therapies with antithymocyte globulin alone and in combination with prednisone or cyclosporine show response rates between 25 and 40% [75, 76].

The studies discussed in this and other chapters of this book will help to translate our knowledge of genetic aberrations and of pathophysiological mechanisms in MDS into clinical use in diagnosis, prognosis, and therapy. Novel agents developed on the basis of this knowledge (luspatercept, rigosertib, immune checkpoint inhibitors, venetoclax, and others) are in clinical trials and will help in relapsed/refractory MDS.

The work of our group in this area was supported by the research project for conceptual development of research organization (00023736; Institute of Hematology and Blood Transfusion, Prague) from the Ministry of Health of the Czech Republic.

Author details

Ota Fuchs
Institute of Hematology and Blood Transfusion, Prague, Czech Republic

*Address all correspondence to: ota.fuchs@uhkt.cz

References

[1] Bejar R, Steensma DP. Recent developments in myelodysplastic syndromes. Blood. 2014;**124**(18):2793-2803. DOI: 10.1182/blood-2014-04-522136

[2] Pellagatti A, Boultwood J. The molecular pathogenesis of the myelodysplastic syndromes. European Journal of Haematology. 2015;**95**(1):3-15. DOI: 10.1111/ejh.12515

[3] Shastri A, Will B, Steidl U, Verma A. Stem and progenitor cell alterations in myelodysplastic syndromes. Blood. 2017;**129**(12):1586-1594. DOI: 10.1182/blood-2016-10-696062

[4] Nazha A, Sekeres MA. Precision medicine in myelodysplastic syndromes and leukemias: Lessons from sequential mutations. Annual Review of Medicine. 2017;**68**:127-137. DOI: 10.1146/annurev-med-062915-095637

[5] Nazha A. The MDS genomics-prognosis symbiosis. Hematology. American Society of Hematology. Education Program. 2018:270-276. DOI: 10.1182/asheducation-2018.1.270

[6] Barreyro L, Chlon TM, Starczynowski DT. Chronic immune response dysregulation in MDS pathogenesis. Blood. 2018;**132**(15):1553-1560. DOI: 10.1182/blood-2018-03-784116

[7] Ganguly BB, Kadam NN. Mutations of myelodysplastic syndromes (MDS): An update. Mutation Research, Reviews in Mutation Research. 2016;**769**:47-62. DOI: 10.1016/j.mrrev.2016.04.009

[8] Gill H, Leung AY, Kwong YL. Molecular and cellular mechanisms of myelodysplastic syndrome: Implications on targeted therapy. International Journal of Molecular Sciences. 2016;**17**(4):440. DOI: 10.3390/ijms17040440

[9] Weinberg OK, Hasserjian RP. The current approach to the diagnosis of myelodysplastic syndromes. Seminars in Hematology. 2019;**56**(1):15-21. DOI: 10.1053/j. seminhematol.2018.05.015

[10] Schanz J, Cevik N, Fonatsch C, Braulke F, Shirneshan K, Bacher U, et al. Detailed analysis of clonal evolution and cytogenetic evolution patterns in patients with myelodysplastic syndromes (MDS) and related myeloid disorders. Blood Cancer Journal. 2018;**8**(3):28. DOI: 10.1038/s41408-018-0061-z

[11] Steensma DP. Clinical consequences of clonal hematopoiesis of indeterminate potential. Blood Advances. 2018;**2**(22):3404-3410. DOI: 10.1182/bloodadvances. 2018020222

[12] Valent P. ICUS, IDUS, CHIP and CCUS: Diagnostic criteria, separation from MDS and clinical implications. Pathobiology. 2019;**86**(1):30-38. DOI: 10.1159/000489042

[13] Patnaik MM, Tefferi A. Refractory anemia with ring sideroblasts (RARS) and RARS with thrombocytosis (RARS-T): 2017 update on diagnosis, risk-stratification, and management. American Journal of Hematology. 2017;**92**(3):297-310. DOI: 10.1002/ajh.24637

[14] Patnaik MM, Tefferi A. Refractory anemia with ring sideroblasts (RARS) and RARS with thrombocytosis (RARS-T)—"2019 update on diagnosis, risk-stratification, and management". American Journal of Hematology. 2019. DOI: 10.1002/ajh.25397

[15] Nikpour M, Scharenberg C, Liu A, Conte S, Karimi M, Mortera-Blanco T, et al. The role of the iron transporter ABCB7 in refractory anemia with ring sideroblasts. Leukemia. 2013;**27**(4):889-896. DOI: 10.1038/leu.2012.298

[16] Nishiyama T, Ishikawa Y, Kawashima N, Akashi A, Adachi Y, Hattori H, et al. Mutation analysis of therapy-related myeloid neoplasms. Cancer Genetics. 2018;**222-223**:38-45. DOI: 10.1016/j.cancergen.2018.02.006

[17] Valka J, Vesela J, Votavova H, Dostalova-Merkerova M, Horakova Z, Campr V, et al. Differential expression of homologous recombination DNA repair genes in the early and advanced stages of myelodysplastic syndrome. European Journal of Haematology. 2017;**99**(4): 323-331. DOI: 10.1111/ejh.12920

[18] Ribeiro HL Jr, Maia ARS, de Oliveira RTG, Dos Santos AWA, Costa MB, Farias IR, et al. Expression of DNA repair genes is important molecular findings in CD34+ stem cells of myelodysplastic syndrome. European Journal of Haematology. 2018;**100**(1):108-109. DOI: 10.1111/ejh.12966

[19] Boultwood J, Pellagatti A, McKenzie AN, Wainscoat JS. Advances in the 5q− syndrome. Blood. 2010;**116**(26):5803-5811. DOI: 10.1182/blood-2010-04-273771

[20] Starczynowski DT, Kuchenbauer F, Argiropoulos B, Sung S, Morin R, Muranyi A, et al. Identification of miR-145 and miR-146a as mediators of the 5q− syndrome phenotype. Nature Medicine. 2010;**16**(1):49-58. DOI: 10.1038/nm.2054

[21] Ebert BL. Molecular dissection of the 5q deletion in myelodysplastic syndrome. Seminars in Oncology. 2011;**38**(5):621-626. DOI: 10.1053/j.seminoncol.2011.04.010

[22] Kumar MS, Narla A, Nonami A, Mullally A, Dimitrova N, Ball B, et al. Coordinate loss of a microRNA and protein-coding gene cooperate in the pathogenesis of 5q− syndrome. Blood. 2011;**118**(17):4666-4673. DOI: 10.1182/blood-2010-12-324715

[23] Fuchs O. Important genes in the pathogenesis of 5q− syndrome and their connection with ribosomal stress and the innate immune system pathway. Leukemia Research and Treatment. 2012;**2012**:179402. DOI: 10.1155/2012/179402

[24] Neuwirtova R, Fuchs O, Holicka M, Vostry M, Kostecka A, Hajkova H, et al. Transcription factors Fli1 and EKLF in the differentiation of megakaryocytic and erythroid progenitor in 5q− syndrome and in Diamond-Blackfan anemia. Annals of Hematology. 2013;**92**(1):11-18. DOI: 10.1007/s00277-012-1568-1

[25] Komrokji RS, Padron E, Ebert BL, List AF. Deletion 5q MDS: Molecular and therapeutic implications. Best Practice & Research. Clinical Haematology. 2013;**26**(4):365-375. DOI: 10.1016/j.beha.2013.10.013

[26] Giagounidis A, Mufti GJ, Fenaux P, Germing U, List A, MacBeth KJ. Lenalidomide as a disease-modifying agent in patients with del(5q) myelodysplastic syndromes: Linking mechanism of action to clinical outcomes. Annals of Hematology. 2014;**93**(1):1-11. DOI: 10.1007/s00277-013-1863-5

[27] List AF, Bennett JM, Sekeres MA, Skikne B, Fu T, Shammo JM, et al. Extended survival and reduced risk of AML progression in erythroid-responsive lenalidomide-treated patients with lower-risk del(5q) MDS. Leukemia. 2014;**28**(5):1033-1040. DOI: 10.1038/leu.2013.305

[28] Pellagatti A, Boultwood J. Recent advances in the 5q− syndrome. Mediterranean Journal of Hematology and Infectious Diseases. 2015;7(1):e2015037. DOI: 10.4084/MJHID.2015.037

[29] Varney ME, Niederkorn M, Konno H, Matsumura T, Gohda J, Yoshida N,

et al. Loss of Tifab, a del(5q) MDS gene, alters hematopoiesis through derepression of Toll-like receptor-TRAF6 signaling. The Journal of Experimental Medicine. 2015;**212**(11):1967-1985. DOI: 10.1084/jem.20141898

[30] Fink EC, Ebert BL. The novel mechanism of lenalidomide activity. Blood. 2015;**126**(21):2366-2369. DOI: 10.1182/blood-2015-07-567958

[31] Guirguis AA, Ebert BL. Lenalidomide: Deciphering mechanisms of action in myeloma, myelodysplastic syndrome and beyond. Current Opinion in Cell Biology. 2015;**37**:61-67. DOI: 10.1016/j.ceb.2015.10.004

[32] Komrokji RS, List AF. Short- and long-term benefits of lenalidomide treatment in patients with lower-risk del(5q) myelodysplastic syndromes. Annals of Oncology. 2016;**27**(1):62-68. DOI: 10.1093/annonc/mdv488

[33] Talati C, Sallman D, List A. Lenalidomide: Myelodysplastic syndromes with del(5q) and beyond. Seminars in Hematology. 2017;**54**(3):159-166. DOI: 10.1053/j.seminhematol.2017. 06.003

[34] Fenaux P, Giagounidis A, Selleslag D, Beyne-Rauzy O, Mittelman M, Muus P, et al. Clinical characteristics and outcomes according to age in lenalidomide-treated patients with RBC transfusion-dependent lower-risk MDS and del(5q). Journal of Hematology & Oncology. 2017;**10**(1):131. DOI: 10.1186/s13045-017-0491-2

[35] Lee JH, List A, Sallman DA. Molecular pathogenesis of myelodysplastic syndromes with deletion 5q. European Journal of Haematology. 2018. DOI: 10.1111/ejh.13207

[36] Ebert BL, Pretz J, Bosco J, Chang CY, Tamayo P, Galili N, et al. Identification of RPS14 as a 5q− syndrome gene by RNA interference screen. Nature. 2008;**451**(7176):335-339. DOI: 10.1038/nature06494

[37] Schneider RK, Schenone M, Ferreira MV, Kramann R, Joyce CE, Hartigan C, et al. Rps14 haploinsufficiency causes a block in erythroid differentiation mediated by S100A8 and S100A9. Nature Medicine. 2016;**22**(3):288-297. DOI: 10.1038/nm.4047

[38] Cluzeau T, McGraw KL, Irvine B, Masala E, Ades L, Basiorka AA, et al. Pro-inflammatory proteins S100A9 and tumor necrosis factor-α suppress erythropoietin elaboration in myelodysplastic syndromes. Haematologica. 2017;**102**(12): 2015-2020. DOI: 10.3324/haematol. 2016. 158857

[39] Vlachos A, Farrar JE, Atsidaftos E, Muir E, Narla A, Markello TC, et al. Diminutive somatic deletions in the 5q region lead to a phenotype atypical of classical 5q− syndrome. Blood. 2013;**122**(14):2487-2490. DOI: 10.1182/blood-2013-06-509935

[40] Czibere A, Bruns I, Junge B, Singh R, Kobbe G, Haas R, et al. Low RPS14 expression is common in myelodysplastic syndromes without 5q− aberration and defines a subgroup of patients with prolonged survival. Haematologica. 2009;**94**(10):1453-1455. DOI: 10.3324/haematol.2009.008508

[41] Wu L, Li X, Xu F, Zhang Z, Chang C, He Q. Low RPS14 expression in MDS without 5q− aberration confers higher apoptosis rate of nucleated erythrocytes and predicts prolonged survival and possible response to lenalidomide in lower risk non-5q− patients. European Journal of Haematology. 2013;**90**(6): 486-493. DOI: 10.1111/ejh.12105

[42] Wei S, Chen X, Rocha K, Epling-Burnette PK, Djeu JY, Liu Q , et al. A critical role for phosphatase

haplodeficiency in the selective suppression of deletion 5q MDS by lenalidomide. Proceedings of the National Academy of Sciences of the United States of America. 2009;**106**(31):12974-12979. DOI: 10.1073/pnas.0811267106

[43] Wei S, Chen X, McGraw K, Zhang L, Komrokji R, Clark J, et al. Lenalidomide promotes p53 degradation by inhibiting MDM2 auto-ubiquitination in myelodysplastic syndrome with chromosome 5q deletion. Oncogene. 2013;**32**(9):1110-1120. DOI: 10.1038/onc. 2012.139

[44] Gandhi AK, Kang J, Naziruddin S, Parton A, Schafer PH, Stirling DI. Lenalidomide inhibits proliferation of Namalwa CSN.70 cells and interferes with Gab1 phosphorylation and adaptor protein complex assembly. Leukemia Research. 2006;**30**(7):849-858

[45] Matsuoka A, Tochigi A, Kishimoto M, Nakahara T, Kondo T, Tsujioka T, et al. Lenalidomide induces cell death in an MDS-derived cell line with deletion of chromosome 5q by inhibition of cytokinesis. Leukemia. 2010;**24**(4):748-755. DOI: 10.1038/leu.2009.296

[46] Venner CP, Woltosz JW, Nevill TJ, Deeg HJ, Caceres G, Platzbecker U, et al. Correlation of clinical response and response duration with miR-145 induction by lenalidomide in CD34(+) cells from patients with del(5q) myelodysplastic syndrome. Haematologica. 2013;**98**(3):409-413. DOI: 10.3324/haematol.2012.066068

[47] Ito T, Ando H, Suzuki T, Ogura T, Hotta K, Imamura Y, et al. Identification of a primary target of thalidomide teratogenicity. Science. 2010;**327**(5971):1345-1350. DOI: 10.1126/science.1177319

[48] Ito T, Handa H. Cereblon and its downstream substrates as molecular targets of immunomodulatory drugs. International Journal of Hematology. 2016;**104**(3):293-299. DOI: 10.1007/s12185-016-2073-4

[49] Chang XB, Stewart AK. What is the functional role of the thalidomide binding protein cereblon? International Journal of Biochemistry and Molecular Biology. 2011;**2**(3):287-294

[50] Kim HK, Ko TH, Nyamaa B, Lee SR, Kim N, Ko KS, et al. Cereblon in health and disease. Pflügers Archiv. 2016;**468**(8):1299-1309. DOI: 10.1007/s00424-016-1854-1

[51] Jonasova A, Bokorova R, Polak J, Vostry M, Kostecka A, Hajkova H, et al. High level of full-length cereblon mRNA in lower risk myelodysplastic syndrome with isolated 5q deletion is implicated in the efficacy of lenalidomide. European Journal of Haematology. 2015;**95**(1):27-34. DOI: 10.1111/ejh.12457

[52] Fischer ES, Böhm K, Lydeard JR, Yang H, Stadler MB, Cavadini S, et al. Structure of the DDB1-CRBN E3 ubiquitin ligase in complex with thalidomide. Nature. 2014;**512**(7512):49-53. DOI: 10.1038/nature13527

[53] Krönke J, Udeshi ND, Narla A, Grauman P, Hurst SN, McConkey M, et al. Lenalidomide causes selective degradation of IKZF1 and IKZF3 in multiple myeloma cells. Science. 2014;**343**(6168):301-305. DOI: 10.1126/science. 1244851

[54] Krönke J, Fink EC, Hollenbach PW, MacBeth KJ, Hurst SN, Udeshi ND, et al. Lenalidomide induces ubiquitination and degradation of CK1α in del(5q) MDS. Nature. 2015;**523**(7559):183-188. DOI: 10.1038/nature14610

[55] Schneider RK, Ademà V, Heckl D, Järås M, Mallo M, Lord AM, et al. Role of casein kinase 1A1 in the biology and targeted therapy of del(5q) MDS. Cancer Cell. 2014;**26**(4):509-520. DOI: 10.1016/j.ccr. 2014.08.001

[56] Smith AE, Kulasekararaj AG, Jiang J, Mian S, Mohamedali A, Gaken J, et al. CSNK1A1 mutations and isolated del(5q) abnormality in myelodysplastic syndrome: A retrospective mutational analysis. The Lancet Haematology. 2015;**2**(5):e212-e221. DOI: 10.1016/S2352-3026(15)00050-2

[57] Heuser M, Meggendorfer M, Cruz MM, Fabisch J, Klesse S, Köhler L, et al. Frequency and prognostic impact of casein kinase 1A1 mutations in MDS patients with deletion of chromosome 5q. Leukemia. 2015;**29**(9):1942-1945. DOI: 10.1038/leu.2015.49

[58] Negoro E, Radiovoyevitch T, Polprasert C, Adema V, Hosono N, Makishima H, et al. Molecular predictors of response in patients with myeloid neoplasms treated with lenalidomide. Leukemia. 2016;**30**(12):2405-2409. DOI: 10.1038/leu.2016.228

[59] Martinez-Høyer S, Mo A, Deng D, Jiang J, Docking R, Li J, et al. Resistance to lenalidomide in del(5q) MDS is mediated by inhibition of drug-induced megakaryocytic differentiation. Blood. 2018;**132**:176. DOI: 10.1182/blood-2018-176

[60] List A, Ebert BL, Fenaux P. A decade of progress in myelodysplastic syndrome with chromosome 5q deletion. Leukemia. 2018;**32**(7):1493-1499. DOI: 10.1038/s41375-018-0029-9

[61] Belickova M, Vesela J, Jonasova A, Pejsova B, Votavova H, Merkerova MD, et al. TP53 mutation variant allele frequency is a potential predictor for clinical outcome of patients with lower-risk myelodysplastic syndromes. Oncotarget. 2016;**7**(24):36266-36279. DOI: 10.18632/oncotarget.9200

[62] Basiorka AA, McGraw KL, De Ceuninck L, Griner LN, Zhang L, Clark JA, et al. Lenalidomide stabilizes the erythropoietin receptor by inhibiting the E3 ubiquitin ligase RNF41. Cancer Research. 2016;**76**(12):3531-3540. DOI: 10.1158/0008-5472.CAN-15-1756

[63] McGraw KL, Fuhler GM, Johnson JO, Clark JA, Caceres GC, Sokol L, et al. Erythropoietin receptor signaling is membrane raft dependent. PLoS One. 2012;**7**(4):e34477. DOI: 10.1371/journal.pone.0034477

[64] McGraw KL, Basiorka AA, Johnson JO, Clark J, Caceres G, Padron E, et al. Lenalidomide induces lipid raft assembly to enhance erythropoietin receptor signaling in myelodysplastic syndrome progenitors. PLoS One. 2014;**9**(12):e114249. DOI: 10.1371/journal.pone.0114249

[65] Komrokji RS, Lancet JE, Swern AS, Chen N, Paleveda J, Lush R, et al. Combined treatment with lenalidomide and epoetin alfa in lower-risk patients with myelodysplastic syndrome. Blood. 2012;**120**(17):3419-3424. DOI: 10.1182/blood-2012-03-415661

[66] Toma A, Kosmider O, Chevret S, Delaunay J, Stamatoullas A, Rose C, et al. Lenalidomide with or without erythropoietin in transfusion-dependent erythropoiesis-stimulating agent-refractory lower-risk MDS without 5q deletion. Leukemia. 2016;**30**(4):897-905. DOI: 10.1038/leu.2015.296

[67] Jonasova A, Neuwirtova R, Polackova H, Siskova M, Stopka T, Cmunt E, et al. Lenalidomide treatment in lower risk myelodysplastic syndromes—The experience of a Czech hematology center. (Positive effect of erythropoietin ± prednisone addition to lenalidomide in refractory or relapsed patients). Leukemia Research. 2018;**69**:12-17. DOI: 10.1016/j.leukres.2018.03.015

[68] Narla A, Dutt S, McAuley JR, Al-Shahrour F, Hurst S, McConkey M, et al. Dexamethasone and

lenalidomide have distinct functional effects on erythropoiesis. Blood. 2011;**118**(8):2296-2304. DOI: 10.1182/blood-2010-11-318543

[69] Komrokji RS, Al Ali NH, Padron E, Cogle C, Tinsley S, Sallman D, et al. Lenalidomide and prednisone in low and intermediate-1 IPSS risk, non-del(5q) MDS patients: A phase II clinical trial. Clinical Lymphoma, Myeloma & Leukemia. 2019. DOI: 10.1016/j.clml.2018.12.014

[70] Basiorka AA, McGraw KL, Eksioglu EA, Chen X, Johnson J, Zhang L, et al. The NLRP3 inflammasome functions as a driver of the myelodysplastic syndrome phenotype. Blood. 2016;**128**(25):2960-2975. DOI: 10.1182/blood-2016-07-730556

[71] Sallman DA, Cluzeau T, Basiorka AA, List A. Unraveling the pathogenesis of MDS: The NLRP3 inflammasome and pyroptosis drive the MDS phenotype. Frontiers in Oncology. 2016;**6**:151. DOI: 10.3389/fonc.2016.00151

[72] Croker BA, Kelliher MA. BID-ding on necroptosis in MDS. Blood. 2019;**133**(2):103-104. DOI: 10.1182/blood-2018-11-886242

[73] Wagner PN, Shi Q, Salisbury-Ruf CT, Zou J, Savona MR, Fedoriw Y, et al. Increased Ripk1-mediated bone marrow necroptosis leads to myelodysplasia and bone marrow failure in mice. Blood. 2019;**133**(2):107-120. DOI: 10.1182/blood-2018-05-847335

[74] Ping Z, Chen S, Hermans SJF, Kenswil KJG, Feyen J, van Dijk C, et al. Activation of NF-κB driven inflammatory programs in mesenchymal elements attenuates hematopoiesis in low-risk myelodysplastic syndromes. Leukemia. 2018. DOI: 10.1038/s41375-018-0267-x

[75] Haider M, Al Ali N, Padron E, Epling-Burnette P, Lancet J, List A, et al. Immunosuppressive therapy: Exploring an underutilized treatment option for myelodysplastic syndrome. Clinical Lymphoma, Myeloma & Leukemia. 2016;**16**(Suppl):S44-S48. DOI: 10.1016/j.clml.2016.02.017

[76] Stahl M, Zeidan AM. Lenalidomide use in myelodysplastic syndromes: Insights into the biologic mechanisms and clinical applications. Cancer. 2017;**123**(10):1703-1713. DOI: 10.1002/cncr.30585

Chapter 2

Diagnosis and Classification of Myelodysplastic Syndrome

Gamal Abdul Hamid, Abdul Wahab Al-Nehmi and Safa Shukry

Abstract

Myelodysplastic syndrome (MDS) is a clonal hematopoietic stem cell disorder characterized by morphological dysplastic changes in one or more of the major hematopoietic cell lines. MDS can present with varying degrees of single or multiple cytopenias including neutropenia, anemia and thrombocytopenia. Presentation of MDS can range from asymptomatic to life threatening. MDS diagnosis and classification present important challenges, particularly in the distinction from benign conditions. French-American-British (FAB) classification proposed a classification based on easily obtainable laboratory information and was recommended in early and as modified by guidelines of new classification of World Health Organization (WHO). The strategy of diagnostic laboratory in MDS depends on morphological changes and is based on existence of dysplastic changes in the peripheral blood and bone marrow including peripheral blood smear, bone marrow aspirate smear and bone marrow trephine biopsy. The correct morphological interpretation and the use of cytogenetics, immunophenotyping, immunohistochemistry and molecular analysis will give valuable information on diagnosis and prognosis.

Keywords: myelodysplasia, cytopenia, diagnostic criteria, classification

1. Introduction

Myelodysplastic syndromes (MDS) are clonal stem cell disorders with a relatively heterogeneous spectrum, characterized by morphological dysplasia in hematopoietic cells and by bone marrow failure and varying degrees of peripheral blood cytopenias. MDS have been recognized for more than 70 years and named refractory anemia, oligoblastic leukemia and smoldering acute leukemia.

The risks of MDS include infection, anemia, bleeding and transformation to acute myeloblastic leukemia (AML) in approximately 30% of cases. MDS incidence increased from less than 5/100,000 for patients less than 60 years to 36.2 per 100,000 in patients more than 80 year old and more common among men.

In the last 20 years, different MDS classification and prognostic scoring systems have been proposed [1]. French-American-British (FAB) classification was recommended in early and as modified by the World Health Organization (WHO). The WHO classification system uses percentages of blasts in bone marrow, ring sideroblasts and dysplastic changes to differentiate MDS subtypes. The International Prognostic Scoring System (IPSS) is based on a multivariate to evaluate the prognosis. The updated and recent scoring system combine with WHO classification for identification transfusion need was modified by Malcovati and co-workers, the so-called WPSS (World Prognostic Scoring System). This score suggests that patients with unilineage erythroid dysplasia do not need transfusion [2].

2. Diagnosis

The risk of MDS increased with advancing age; approximately 86% of patients with newly diagnosed MDS predominate in the elderly, with a median age at diagnosis 65 years [3]. The age of MDS patients at diagnosis was different according to residency; the results of some studies on patients show that the median age of diagnosis in German, Japan, and Korea were 74, 60, and 57 years, respectively [4].

The chosen diagnostic criterion of MDS is the dysplasia in ≥10% of total count, this morphology features can point to underlying pathological cytogenetic changes which suggestive MDS diagnosis according to the World Health Organization (WHO) 2016 revision [5].

The minimal prerequisites diagnostic guidelines for MDS according to an International Working Group (IWG) are: (1) stable cytopenia for >6 months unless accompanied a specific chromosomal analysis (Karyotype) or bilineage dysplasia [6]; (2) the exclusion of other potential disorders as a primary reason for dysplasia or cytopenia or both.

3. Diagnostic workup

MDS diagnosis based on morphological characteristics of bone marrow dysplasia in patients with clinical manifestations evidence of hematopoiesis impairments by different combinations of anemia, leukopenia, neutropenia and thrombocytopenia. The National Comprehensive Cancer Network (NCCN) recommend specific guidelines for evaluation of MDS include physical examination; peripheral blood examination, bone marrow examination with iron stain and cytogenetic, RBC folate and vitamin B12 and serum ferritin [7]. The combination peripheral cytopenias despite of bone marrow hypercellularity is the hallmark of MDS, and is a consequence of bone marrow dysfunction with an increase apoptosis rate of bone marrow cells.

According to NCCN the diagnosis of MDS requires ≥1 of MDS-related criteria: (1) dysplasia (≥10% in ≥1 of bone marrow cell line); (2) presence of 5–19% blast cells; and (3) presence of a specific MDS-linked chromosomal abnormalities like del(5q), del(20q), +8, or −7/del(7q) [8].

4. Differential diagnosis

Before treatment, the major role is to distinguish MDS from other causes of cytopenia and dysplastic changes and from other clonal stem cell disorders [9]. The investigations work-up is important to rule the possible differential diagnosis and pre-MDS conditions (**Table 1**).

4.1 Cytopenic causes

1. Chronic liver diseases

2. Drug induced cytopenia

	Characteristics
IDUS	Mild cytopenias for >6 months (Hb ≥ 11/dl, neutrophils ≥ 1500/μl, platelets ≥ 100,000/μl, all below lower limit of normal) or no cytopenias but marked dysplasia in >10% of cell lineages and no clonal cytogenetic/molecular markers
ICUS	Mild cytopenias (hemoglobin <11.0 g/dl, neutropenia <1500/μl and/or thrombocytopenia <100,000/μl and lack of significant dysplasia in the bone marrow but exclusion of other diseases and/or no clonal cytogenetic/molecular markers
CCUS	Hemoglobin, <11 g/dl, ANC <1500/μl, platelet count <100,000/μl, ≥10% dysplasia in the granulocytic, erythroid, or megakaryocytic lineage, myeloblasts comprise ≥5% of total cellularity. Common mutations; TET2, DNMT3A, ASXL1, SRSF2, TP53
CHIP	The presence of clonal hematopoiesis in the absence of cytopenias and dysplastic changes. The incidence of CHIP increases with age. Common mutations; TET2, DNMT3A, ASXL1, PPM1D, JAK2, TP53, *SF3B1*

ICUS, idiopathic cytopenia of uncertain significance; ICUS, idiopathic dysplasia of unknown significance; CCUS, clonal cytopenia of undetermined significance; CHIP, clonal hematopoiesis of indeterminate potential.
An absence of mutation and unexplained cytopenias are criteria do not meet World Health Organization (WHO)-defined requirements for myelodysplastic syndrome.

Table 1.
Differentiation of ICUS, IDUS, CCUS and CHIP [8].

3. Excessive alcohol intake
4. Cytotoxic therapy
5. B12/folate deficiency
6. Autoimmune cytopenia
7. Anemia of chronic disorders
8. Parasitic manifestation (hypersplenism in malaria and leishmaniasis)
9. Human immunodeficiency virus infection (HIV)
10. Other stem cell disorder

4.2 Idiopathic cytopenia of uncertain significance (ICUS)

4.3 Idiopathic dysplasia of unknown significance (IDUS)

4.4 Clonal cytopenia of undetermined significance (CCUS)

4.5 Clonal hematopoiesis of indeterminate potential (CHIP)

5. Clinical presentation

Clinical presentation of MDS is nonspecific and varies considerably depending on subtypes and severity of cytopenias. This should include family history, tobacco, alcohol intake, pesticides, heavy metals, prior chemotherapy, irradiation, radioiodine, radioimmunotherapy, concomitant medication including "alternative medication", infection, tendency for bleeding/bruising, and a complete physical examination including spleen size. Symptoms can include general weakness, pallor, shortness of breathing, bleeding manifestations; gum bleeding and petechiae.

6. Blood tests

Complete blood count (CBC) includes white blood cell count (WBC) with differential blood count including erythrocyte morphology, hemoglobin, platelet count, red blood cell indices, mean corpuscular volume (MCV), and reticulocyte count.

Serum tests of erythropoietin, protein electrophoresis, folic acid, cobalamin, iron, total iron binding capacity (TIBC), ferritin, lactate dehydrogenase (LDH), bilirubin, Coombs test, alanine aminotransferase (ALT) test, aspartate aminotransferase (AST), alkaline phosphatase, albumin, uric acid, creatinine (S-immunoglobulins), B2 microglobulin and thyroid function tests.

Also some investigations are mandatory to exclude viral infection especially; anti-HIV, anti-Parvovirus B19 (hypoplastic MDS), hepatitis C antibody, hepatitis B surface antigen (HBsAg) and cytomegalovirus test (CMV) in transfusion dependent patients.

Cytogenetic study for BCR-ABL and JAK2 (Janus kinase 2) are important for differential diagnosis of myeloproliferative disorders.

6.1 Interpretation of peripheral blood

The WHO recommendations for the definition of cytopenia are the same reported in the International Prognostic Scoring System (IPSS), when the hemoglobin less than 10 g/dl, the leukocyte count 3000/mm^3, an absolute neutrophil less than 1800/mm^3 and platelets less than 100,000/mm^3. These thresholds have been a matter of debate, and as a result, any cytopenia should be differentiated from MDS in case of clear morphologic or the result of genetic features consistent with MDS [5, 6]. Anemia is represent in most patients, the mean corpuscular volume (MCV) is often increased and an increased erythrocyte distribution width (RDW) which the erythropoiesis disturbances. A dimorphic red blood cell (RBC) population (macrocytes and microcytes), anisocytosis, poikilocytosis, nucleated red blood cells, basophilic stippling and Howell-Jolly bodies are also indications that the erythrocyte has undergone abnormal development [10]. Peripheral blood may reveal very abnormal nuclei such as Pelger-Huet anomalies and hypo-or hypersegmentation and ring forms nuclei also occur in neutrophils are important morphological features in MDS/MPN peripheral blood when diagnosing and distinguishing MDS/MPN is important to understand the similarities and differences in pathologic mechanism from similar diseases (AML, infectious diseases and other causes of cytopenia). The platelet morphological changes include giant platelets and platelets hypogranulation or agranulation. Some platelets may possess large fused granules. Circulating micromegakaryocytes (dwarf cells), multiple small nuclei separated by strands of nuclear material, and large mononuclear cells with dysmorphic nuclear features have been described in peripheral blood from patients with MDS [11].

The diagnosis of MDS requires a careful light microscopic examination of optimally stained peripheral blood and bone marrow smear and trephine biopsy sections with presence of 1% blast in peripheral blood, with <5% BM blasts and uni- or multilineage dysplasia is defined as unclassifiable MDS. Monocytic hyperplasia accounting for >10% of the white blood cells is a common finding in chronic myelomonocytic leukemia (CMML) and is a common finding in dysplastic marrows and can be dominant manifestation of the hematopoietic abnormality in CMML for months and years.

Cell line	Peripheral blood	Bone marrow
Erythroid	Dimorphic; macrocytic; anisocytosis; polychromatic; hypochromasia, tear drop cells Pappenheimer bodies; basophilic stippling	Erythroid hyperplasia; megaloblastic changes; dyserythropoiesis; multinuclearity, nuclear bridges, nuclear budding, atypical mitosis, ring sideroblasts
Granulocytes	Hypersegmented neutrophils; hypogranular or agranular neutrophils; pseudo-Pelger cells	Shift to left, promyelocytes with absent or spares azurophilic granules; hypogranular myelocytes, metamyelocytes and neutrophils, Auer rods, pseudo-Pelger cells, nuclear anomalies
Monocytes	Mature monocytes	Increase and morphological abnormalities of monocytes
Megakaryocytes	Thrombocytosis; giant platelets	Increase or decrease; mononuclear megakaryocytes, micromegakaryocytes, hypersegmented megakaryocytes
Blasts	**Figure 2**	

The highly specific dysplastic changes in granulocytes of patients with MDS are hypoagranularity and nuclear abnormality of neutrophils in peripheral blood smear and positive on peroxidase reaction or Sudan black. The highly specific dysplastic changes in erythropoiesis are sideroblastic rings and megaloblastoid changes. The highly specific for dysmegakaryopoiesis are micromegakaryocytes.

Table 2.
MDS morphology abnormalities on peripheral blood and bone marrow [12, 13].

7. Bone marrow aspirate and biopsy

A diagnosis of MDS often requires repeated bone marrow aspiration/biopsy examinations a few weeks or months, or even years apart in order to firmly establish the diagnosis and to identify cases with rapid disease progression. Bone marrow morphology evaluation and dysplasia in blood and bone marrow follow guidelines in the WHO 2016 classification. A good quality diagnostic bone marrow analysis includes marrow aspirate May-Grunewald Giemsa (MGG)/equivalent and bone marrow iron stain and a bone marrow biopsy either decalcified/paraffin embedded or plastic embedded. Degree of fibrosis should be estimated. The cytochemistry staining should include iron staining, Peroxidase-Staining, in addition to hematoxylin-eosin/equivalent [12].

The cell counting of bone marrow and blood smear should include at least 200 cells in blood smear, 500 cells in bone marrow and 25 megakaryocytes and at least 100 erythroblasts should be evaluated. An optimal staining of blood and marrow slides prepared from freshly drawn aspirates is important for evaluation of dysplasia (**Table 2**) [12–15].

8. Dysplastic features

Dysplastic changes are the most important diagnostic features of myelodysplastic syndrome. A marrow cell lineage is considered picture of MDS if >10% of cells are affected.

8.1 Dyserythropoiesis

Dyserythropoiesis is the presence of oval macrocytes and erythroblast may resemble megaloblasts that have nuclear-cytoplasmic maturation asynchrony, nuclear fragmentation, or cytoplasmic nuclear remnants. This pattern is referred to as megaloblastoid erythropoiesis [14–16]. A dimorphic red blood cell population,

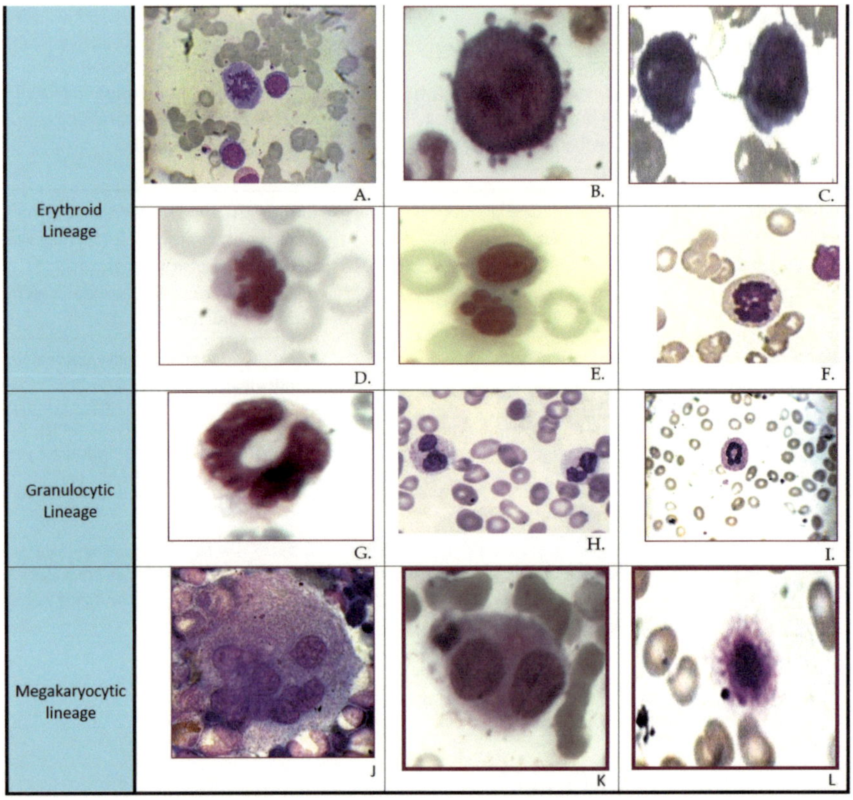

Figure 1.
Morphological abnormalities of myelodysplastic syndrome: Leishman stain. (I) Erythroid dysplastic changes; (A) megaloblastic changes, (B) cytoplasmic fraying, (C) internuclear bridging, (D) nuclear lobulation, (E) nuclear lobulation (F) karyorrhexis (II) granulocytic dysplastic changes; (G) hypogranulation band neutrophil, (H) pseudo-Pelger anomaly, (I) nucleus ring or doughnut shaped (III) megakaryocytic dysplastic changes; (J) hypersegmented, (k) micromegakaryocyte, (L) giant abnormal platelet.

anisocytosis, poikilocytosis, nucleated red blood cells, Howell-Jolly bodies and basophilic stippling are indications that the erythrocyte has undergone abnormal development. The RBC with abnormally round nucleus may have lobes or buds, internuclear bridging, nuclear fragments and abnormal mitosis are occasionally present. Pathologic sideroblast may be identified when the marrow treated with Prussian blue stain (**Figure 1**) [14, 15].

8.2 Dysmyelopoiesis

The most striking abnormalities are hypogranulated neutrophils. The defect in granulation may be seen in myelocytes early in the course of disease. Very abnormal nuclei, such as Pelger-Huet anomalies and hypo- or hypergranulation, and ring shaped nuclei in neutrophils. Monocytic hyperplasia is a common finding in dysplastic marrows and can be the dominant manifestation of the hematopoietic abnormalities of CMML for months or years (**Figure 1**) [11]. Cytoplasmic changes may include uneven staining such as a dense ring of basophilia around the periphery with a clear unstained area around the nucleus [14, 15]. Occasionally there are Auer rods, either in circulating or BM blast cells, entails an unfavorable prognosis and this could lead to misclassification the disease in the AML. Myeloperoxidase and the study of specific immunophenotypic markers are helpful to differentiate between MDS and other types of AML [17].

8.3 Dysmegakaryopoiesis

The common changes include giant platelets and abnormal platelet granulation, either hypogranulation or agranulation. Some platelets may possess large fused granules. Circulating micromegakaryocytes, multiple small nuclei separated by stands of nuclear material and large mononuclear cell with dysmorphic nuclear features have been described in peripheral blood of patients with MDS (**Figure 1**) [13–15].

For significant dysplasia, dysplastic features should be present in at least 10% of the nucleated cells in the lineage in consideration.

9. Blast cells

9.1 Counting blasts

Myeloblast cell should be differentiated from promyelocyte. The promyelocyte is larger than myeloblast and characterized by clear Golgi zone and azurophilic granulations. Myeloblast was defined in terms of several nuclear characteristics, including a high nuclear/cytoplasmic ratio, easily visible nucleoli and usually contain fine nuclear chromatin and viable nuclear shape. The International Working Group (IWGM) recommended that myeloblast in MDS should be classified as agranular or granular [12]. The agranular blast corresponds to the type I blast of the FAB classification. Type II have scanty granules [18] and type III blast with more than 20 fine azurophilic granules as defined by Goasguen et al. [13]. The nuclear characteristic of promyelocytes included an eccentric or central nucleus and intermediate or fine chromatin and azurophilic granulation (**Figure 2**) [12].

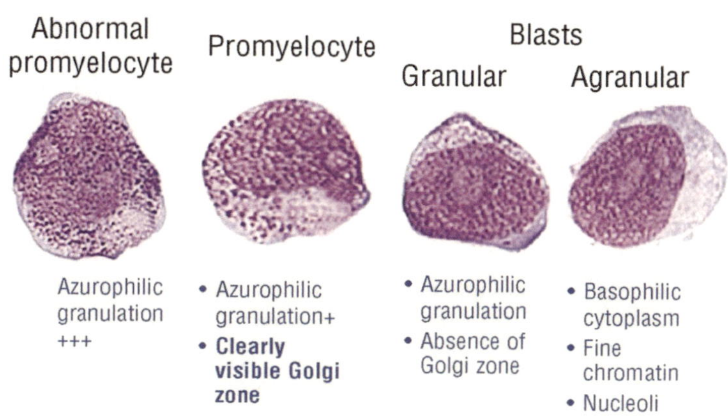

Figure 2.
Blasts, promyelocytes, abnormal promyelocytes, modified of Mufti et al. [12]. In MDS, the granular and agranular blasts have azurophilic granules and Auer rods; both exhibit visible nucleoli, scant basophilic cytoplasm, lack Golgi zone and exist of fine nuclear chromatin, while promyelocytes have eccentric nucleus with visible nucleoli and Golgi zone and exist of azurophilic granules.

10. Cytogenetic analysis

The cytogenetic study of bone marrow aspirate has a major role in determining clonality in patients with MDS. Karyotyping should be done in all patients, at least 25 metaphases, whenever possible, and described according to International System recommendations. Chromosomal abnormalities are reported in more

Prognostic category	Chromosomal categories	Median survival (months)
Very good	Del(11q), −Y	60
Good	Normal, del(5q), double aberrations including del(5q), del(12p), del (20q)	40.5
Intermediate	Del(7q), +8.i(17q), +19, any other	25.0
Poor	Inv(3)/t(3q), −7, −7/7q, double aberrations including −7/7q−, complex karyotypes with 3 abnormalities	15.0
Very poor	Complex karyotypes with >3 abnormalities	5.7

IPSS-R, Revised International Prognostic Scoring System.
MDS prognosis is calculated by utilizing the International Prognostic Scoring System (IPSS) score, which includes cytogenetics analyzed categories, in addition to number of cytopenias and counting of blast percentage. The present of >3 chromosomal abnormalities indicate very poor prognosis.

Table 3.
Cytogenetic prognosis in MDS according IPSS-R [21, 22].

than 50% of patients with MDS by counting 25 metaphase cytogenetic analysis, but not by fluorescence in situ hybridization (FISH) or sequencing technologies. The technique by using FISH method may be helpful to detect monosomy 7 and to clarify complex aberrations. Screening FISH (5q−, −7, +8) from peripheral blood may be performed in patients of dry tap bone marrow and this may influence management of the patient [19]. Different cytogenetic abnormalities are considered MDS-defining [20]. The presence monosomy 5, 7, or 13; 5q, 7q and 13q deletions; i(17p) and t(17p); 11q deletion; 9q or 12p deletion or t(12p), idic (X)(q13) allows for the diagnosis of MDS even in the absence of dysplastic changes. Cytogenetic is strongly correlated with not only the calculation prognosis but also selection of the most effective therapy; thus, a complete BM karyotype remains the standard work up evaluation procedure of the patient with MDS according to IPSS-R (**Table 3**) [21, 22].

11. Molecular genetic testing

The most important mutated genes for MDS prognostication involved in epigenetic regulation are acquired mutation have been detected in several genes: (*ASXL1, EZH2, DNMT3A, TET2, IDH1/2, pre-mRNA* splicing factors *(SF3B1, SRSF2, U2AF1) transcription (RUNX1, TP53*) and signaling transduction are seen in MDS and can demonstrate clonal disease [23]. According to the new *2016* World Health Organization (WHO) Classification of MDS, the analysis of the SF3B1 considered the only important diagnostic method for diagnosis of MDS-RS. The prognosis of MDS-RS is favorable in presence of SF3B1 mutations [24]. Mutations in the ASXL1, TP53, ETV6, RUNX1 and EZH2 are reported as independently associated with decreased overall survival in cases of MDS [25].

12. Immunophenotyping

By flow cytometry and immunohistochemistry, immunophenotyping of the blast population can be useful for emerging pathological CD34 and or CD117 and myeloperoxidase (MPO) positive populations are suggestive of transformation.

According to WHO classification 2016, the best method for diagnosis of MDS is the percentages of blast cells in bone marrow. The immunophenotyping can be useful to study the expression of maturation and anomalies as marker of dysplasia of a particular lineage [26].

Multiple aberrant features (>3) in maturation patterns of erythroid and myeloid lineage are highly specific for MDS, but single aberrancies are not diagnostic [27]. The role of flow cytometry can be useful in the diagnostic work-up of MDS, and to detect minimal residual disease after treatment according to the European Leukemia Net (ELN) work package for flow cytometry [28]. For prognostic follow up, the increase expression of CD33, CD34, CD13, HLA-DR/human leukocyte antigen-DR and decreased reactivity for CD11b in the bone marrow have been associated with shorter survival and high risk of transformation to acute leukemia.

13. Classification

13.1 FAB classification

Several classifications have been developed to predict the transformation of MDS to acute myeloid leukemia (AML). In 1982, the FAB system, was introduced based on percentage of blasts and morphological features in blood and bone marrow, namely medullary and peripheral blast cell count, ringed sideroblasts, number of monocytes in peripheral blood, and Auer rods. According to this classification, patients are diagnosed with MDS when dysplastic changes in bone marrow are present and/or myeloblast cells are between 5 and 30% of all bone marrow cells. Five subgroups with significantly different prognoses were established: refractory anemia (RA) with blasts <5% in BM, refractory anemia with ringed sideroblasts (RARS) with blasts <5% and ring sideroblasts >15%, refractory anemia with excess of blasts between 5 and 20% (RAEB), RAEB in transformation to acute leukemia and blast cells ranged between 20 and 30% (RAEB-T) and chronic myelomonocytic leukemia characterized by increase of peripheral blood monocytes (CMML) (**Table 4**) [20, 29]. For more than 20 years this classification served as the standard for the evaluation of MDS [30]. Hypercellular MDS, and MDS with bone marrow fibrosis were not recognized by the FAB classification [31].

Type	Blasts in blood	Blasts in bone marrow
1. Refractory anemia (RA)	<1%	Blasts <5%, ring sideroblastic <15%
2. Refractory anemia with ring sideroblastic (RARS)	<1%	Blasts <5%, ring sideroblasts >15%
3. Refractory anemia with excess of blast (RAEB)	<5%	Blasts 5–20%
4. Refractory anemia with excess blast in transformation (RAEB-t)	<30%	Blasts 20–30%
5. Chronic myelomonocytic leukemia (CMMoL)	<5% with increase monocytes	Blasts 0–20%
AML	>30%	>30%

Modified of Ref. [20].
CMML, chronic myelomonocytic leukemia blast cells <20% and monocytes ≥1000/μl); RA, refractory anemia <1% in PB and <5% blasts in BM; RAEB, RA with excess blasts in PB <5% and 5–20% blasts in BM; RAEB-t, RAEB with excess blasts in transformation between 20 and 30%; RARS, RA with ringed sideroblasts >15%.

Table 4.
Myelodysplastic syndrome (MDS) according to FAB classification [20].

13.2 WHO classification

The World Health Organization (WHO) classification of MDS revised in 1999 and redefine subtypes of MDS [32]. The definitions of refractory anemia (RA) and refractory anemia with ring sideroblastic (RARS) unchanged became more consistent and characterized by the presence of dysplastic morphology in the erythroid cell line. Refractory anemia with ring sideroblastic (RARS) is morphologically similar to *RA* with the presence of ≥15% ring sideroblasts.

Refractory anemia with excess of blasts (RAEB) recognized by the World Health Organization (WHO) classification in all versions and remains unchanged but distinguishes between two categories of RAEB: RAEB-1 with 5–10% blast cells and RAEB-2 with 11–20% blasts in the bone marrow.

The other new subgroups of MDS were incorporated: (1) refractory cytopenia with multilineage dysplasia (RC1Dys), is a frequent subtype of MDS, which is equivalent to RA or RARS in the FAB classification with the presence of dysplasia but lacking an increase in blast cells with no Auer rods or increase of monocytes; (2) del (5q) syndrome is a myelodysplastic disorder characterized by macrocytic anemia, dysplastic changes in the erythroid cell line only, thrombocytosis and increase of hypolobulated micromegakaryocyte; (3) MDS unclassifiable; myelodysplastic syndromes that do not meet criteria of a specific WHO entity.

RAEB-T and CMML subgroups were removed from the new MDS classification: RAEB-T, because of distinctive biologic features and similarities in treatment strategies with acute myeloid leukemia (AML), and CMML, because of having overlapping dysplastic and proliferative features and its close relation to myeloproliferative diseases [33].

2008 WHO classification	2016 WHO classification
Refractory cytopenia with unilineage dysplasia (RCUD) encompassing refractory anemia (RA), refractory neutropenia (RN), and refractory thrombocytopenia (RT)	MDS with single lineage dysplasia (MDS-SLD)
Refractory cytopenia with multilineage dysplasia (RCMD)	MDS with multilineage dysplasia (MDS-MLD)
Refractory anemia with ringed sideroblasts (RARS)	**MDS with ring sideroblasts (MDS-RS)**
	MDS-RS with single lineage dysplasia (MDS-RS-SLD)
	MDS-RS with multilineage dysplasia (MDS-RS-MLD)
Myelodysplastic syndrome associated with isolated del(5q)	MDS with isolated del(5q)
	MDS with excess blasts (MDS-EB)
Refractory anemia with excess blasts-1 (RAEB-1)	MDS-EB-1
Refractory anemia with excess blasts-2 (RAEB-2)	MDS-EB-2
Myelodysplastic syndrome, unclassified (MDS-U)	**MDS, unclassifiable (MDS-U)**
	With 1% blood blasts
	With single lineage dysplasia and pancytopenia
	Based on defining cytogenetic abnormality
Refractory cytopenia of childhood	Refractory cytopenia of childhood

WHO, World Health Organization; MDS, myelodysplastic syndromes; RS, ring sideroblasts; RCUD, refractory cytopenia with unilineage dysplasia; RCMD, refractory cytopenia with multilineage dysplasia; MDS-MLD, MDS with multilineage dysplasia; MDS-SLD, MDS with single lineage dysplasia; MDS-EB, MDS with excess blasts; MDS-U, MSD, unclassifiable; RCC, refractory cytopenia of childhood.

Table 5.
World Health Organization (WHO) classifications of myelodysplastic syndromes [20, 22].

In 2001, the WHO proposed an alternative classification for MDS that was modified from the original French-American-British (FAB) definitions [18]. Since then, the WHO classification has been updated twice (2008 and 2016) (**Table 5**) [22, 33].

The last edition of WHO classification guidelines identify 6 types of MDS: MDS with single lineage dysplasia (MDS-SLD); MDS with ring sideroblasts (MDS-RS); MDS with multilineage dysplasia; MDS with excess blasts (MDS-EB); MDS with isolated del(5q); and MDS unclassifiable (MDS-U). There is an additional provisional entity termed "refractory cytopenia of childhood." MDS-SLD includes refractory anemia (unilineage erythroid dysplasia), refractory neutropenia (unilineage dysgranulopoiesis), and refractory thrombocytopenia (unilineage dysmegakaryocytopoiesis). The latter 2 were previously classified as MDS-U in 2001 but were reclassified in the 2008 update [34].

According to 2016 WHO classification guidelines identify MDS subtypes based on the results of blood and bone marrow test. The classification of 2016 WHO of MDS was according to factors that differ from those of the FAB system and defined by precise criteria including: (1) dysplastic changes (2) number of cytopenia in peripheral blood (3) percentage of sideroblastic rings (**Table 6**) [5].

13.2.1 MDS with single lineage dysplasia (MDS-SLD)

One dysplastic lineage with dysplasia in at least 10% of the early cells of 2 or 3 cell types (red blood cells, white blood cells, and/or megakaryocytes in the bone marrow. No Auer rodes blast cells less than 5% in BM and <1% in PB. Sideroblastic ring less than 15% in BM and <5% in PB.

Subtype	Blood	Bone marrow
(1) MDS with single lineage dysplasia (MDS-SLD)	Single of bicytopenia	Dysplasia in ≥10 of one cell line, <5% blasts
(2) MDS with ring sideroblasts (MDS-RS)	Anemia, no blasts	≥15% of erythroid precursors w/ ring sideroblasts, or ≥5% of ring sideroblasts, <5% blasts
(3) MDS with multilineage dysplasia (MDS-MLD)	Cytopenia(s*), <1 or 10^9/l monocytes	Dysplasia in ≥10 of cells in ≥2 hematopoietic lineages, ±15% ring sideroblasts, <5% blasts
(4.1) MDS with excess blasts-1 (MDS-EB-1)	Cytopenia(s), ≤2–4% blasts#, <1 × 10^9/l monocytes	Unilineage or multilineage dysplasia, 5–9% blasts, no Auer rods
(4.2) MDS with excess blasts-2 (MDS-EB-2)	Cytopenia(s), 5–19% blasts#, <1 × 10^9/l monocytes	Unilineage or multilineage dysplasia, 10–19% blasts, ±Auer rods
(5) MDS with isolated del(5q)	Anemia, platelets normal or increased	Unilineage erythroid dysplasia, isolated del(5q), <5% blasts
(6) MDS, unclassifiable (MDS-U)	Cytopenia(s), +1% blasts on at least 2 occasions	Unilineage dysplasia or no dysplasia but characteristic MDS cytogenetics, <5% blasts
(7) Refractory cytopenia of childhood	Cytopenias, <2% blasts	Dysplasia in 1–3 lineages, <5% blasts

**Cytopenias defined as: hemoglobin, 10 g/dl; absolute neutrophil count, 1800/mm^3 and platelet count less than 100,000/mm^3; S; bicytopenia may be observed in most cases of MDS.*
#Present of 5–9% myeloblast in BM and 2–4% myeloblasts in the blood, the diagnostic is MDS-EB-1 and 10–19% myeloblast in BM and 5–19% myeloblasts in the blood, the diagnostic is MDS-EB-2. Cases with pancytopenia with unilineage or absent dysplasia with 1% myeloblasts in the blood should be classified as MDS-U.

Table 6.
Peripheral blood and bone marrow findings according to 2016 WHO classification of MDS [5, 20].

13.2.2 MDS with ring sideroblasts (MDS-RS)

MDS-RS previously named as refractory anemia with ring sideroblasts (RARS). In this type of MDS, there is increased sideroblastic rings of nucleated red blood and for diagnosis, ring sideroblasts seen in nucleated red blood cells or at least 5% if the cells also have high of *SF3B1* mutations [35]. Mutations in SF3B1 are seen in ≥80% of cases.

MDS-RS include 2 subtypes based on dysplastic bone marrow:

- MDS-RS with single lineage dysplasia (MDS-RS-SLD): one dysplastic lineage, one or two PB cytopenia, sideroblastic rings >15% in BM or 5% in cases with SF3B1 mutation, blast cells <5% in BM and <1% in PB and no Auer rods.

- MDS-RS with multilineage dysplasia (MDS-RS-MLD): dysplasia in more than one lineage, one to three PB cytopenias, sideroblastic ring in BM 15 and 5% if SF3B1 mutation is present. Blast cells in BM <5% and in PB <1% without Auer rods.

This type of MDS is not common. It rarely turns into AML, and the outcome for people with this type is generally better than for some other types of MDS.

13.2.3 MDS with multilineage dysplasia (MDS-MLD)

Dysplastic changes in two or three lineages and PB cytopenia in one to three lineages, sideroblastic ring in 15% in BM or 5% in cases with SF3B1 mutation, blast cell without Auer rods <5% in BM and <1% in PB.

13.2.4 MDS with excess blasts (MDS-EB)

In this type of MDS, the blasts are present in the bone marrow and/or peripheral blood. Dysplastic changes present in one to three lineage and cytopenia in one to three lines. Sideroblastic ring not present.

There are 2 types, based on how many of the cells in the bone marrow or blood are blasts:

- *MDS* with excess blasts-1 (MDS-EB1): *blast* cells make up 5–9% in the bone marrow aspirate, or 2–4% of blast cells in peripheral blood and absent of Auer rods.

- *MDS* with excess blasts-2 (MDS-EB2): previously named *refractory anemia with excess blasts* (RAEB), characterized by excess blasts 10–19% of bone marrow aspirate cells, or 5–19% blast cells in peripheral blood and/or present of Auer rods.

13.2.5 MDS with isolated del(5q)

"5q– syndrome" is a specific type of myelodysplastic syndrome (MDS). Is not common and it occurs most often in older women. It is characterized by missing part of chromosome number 5. The patient also has cytopenia in one or two blood cell lines with common manifestations including severe anemia, typical dysmegakaryopoiesis, frequent thrombocytosis and favorable outcome [5]. The median survival of patients with isolated 5q– syndrome of 9 years and they have good prognosis and rarely transform to develop AML [35].

13.2.6 MDS, unclassifiable (MDS-U)

This type of MDS is uncommon. For MDS-U, the pathological findings in bone marrow more than in peripheral blood. We observe that, one or more cytopenias are a standard feature of MDS-U but other clinical features are variable. Dysplastic changes in bone marrow in less than 10% but typical cytogenetic abnormality was reported [5].

13.2.7 Refractory cytopenia of childhood

Usually hypocellular with similar picture of aplastic anemia. The mutations are less common than in adult MDS (24% of patients) and have a different profile NRAS/KRAS, SETBP1, ASXL1, RUNX1, BCOR/BCORL, PTPN.

14. Chronic myelomonocytic leukemia (CMML)

14.1 Definition

Chronic myelomonocytic leukemia (CMML) is a clonal hematopoietic stem cell disorder classified by the WHO as an overlapping feature of myelodysplastic syndromes and myeloproliferative neoplasms (MPN). It is characterized by peripheral blood monocytosis, dysplastic features in at least 1 hematopoietic cell line and increased risk of progression to AML [36].

The disease annual incidence became stable at around 0.4 per 100,000 population in Western countries [37]. CMML is occurring in elderly patients whose median age at diagnosis is 71–75 years. The incidence of CMML was higher in men than in women whose origin remains unclear [37].

14.2 Diagnosis of CMML

Diagnosis is based on the presence of sustained (>3 months) peripheral blood monocytosis ($\geq 1 \times 10^9$/l; monocytes ≥10%), along with bone marrow dysplastic changes. Bone marrow and BCR-ABL are recommended to exclude acute leukemia and a classic myeloproliferative neoplasms. Atypical monocytes differ from promonocytes and monoblasts. They contain no nucleolus, exhibit swelling, abnormally folded nuclei, aggregated chromatin, nucleus-cytoplasm asynchrony. Their presence is usually associated with increase of neutrophils and shift to left picture with increase of platelet count but the association of macrocytic anemia and thrombocytopenia are the most common [38]. The CMML classified into three groups/categories for precise prognostication include: CMML0; a group with <2% blasts in PB and <5% blast in BM, the second group CMML1 include patients with 2–5% blasts in PB and 5–9% blasts in BM and third group include patients with 5–9% blasts in PB and 10–19% blasts in BM (**Table 7**) [5, 39].

14.2.1 Immunophenotyping of CMML

An international nomenclature has been used to help diagnose CMML [40]. Human monocytes can be divided into three subsets; MO1, CD14+/CD16− (classical), MO2, CD14+/CD16+ (intermediate) and MO3, CD14−/CD16+ (nonclassical). CMML is characterized by the accumulation of classical monocytes with an MO1 threshold to 94% of total circulating monocytes and with different gene expression profiles, chemokine receptor expressions and phagocytic activities [41].

Persistent monocytosis ≥1 × 10^9/l and monocytes ≥10% of WBC in peripheral blood
<20% blasts in peripheral blood and bone marrow aspiration*
No criteria and no previous history of CML, ET**, PV, and PMF
If eosinophilia, no *PDGFRA*, *PDGFRB*, *FGFR1* rearrangement, no *PMC1-JAK2* fusion gene
≥1 following criteria: 1. Acquired clonal cytogenetic or molecular abnormality in hematopoietic cells*** 2. Dysplasia in ≥1 myeloid lineage 3. Monocytosis persistent for at least 3 months, with other causes excluded

CML, chronic myeloid leukemia; ET, essential thrombocythemia; PV, polycythemia vera; PMF, primary myelofibrosis; WBC, white blood cell.

**Total blast cells include monoblast, promonoblasts and myeloblasts.*

***Exclude of myeloproliferative neoplasms (MPN) associated with monocytosis by bone marrow cytology and/or of MPN-associated mutations (JAK2, calreticulin gene "CALR", or myeloproliferative leukemia mutation "MPL") tend to confirm the diagnosis of MPN with monocytosis rather than chronic myelomonocytic leukemia (CMML).*
****The mutations associated with CMML which may support confirmation of diagnosis like ASXL1, SRSF2, SETBP1, TET2.*

Table 7.
Diagnostic criteria of CMML modified according to Daniel Arber of 2016 WHO classification Blood 2016 [5].

14.2.2 Cytogenetic abnormalities of CMML

Clonal cytogenetic abnormalities identify non-specific chromosomal abnormalities in 30–40% of CMML patients. Peripheral blood/bone marrow for BCR-ABL rearrangement for all patients should be done to exclude any pathological disorder related to myeloproliferative disorders and PDGFRA, PDGFRB, FGFR1 rearrangements or PCM1-JAK2 (**Table** 7) [5, 42]. The most common alterations include; trisomy 8 (4–11%),—Y (5–20%), abnormalities of chromosome 7 (monosomy 7 and del7q) in 2–14%, trisomy 21, and complex karyotypes [43].

15. Conclusions

Myelodysplastic syndrome diagnosis based on data accumulated since the 2008 WHO classification of MDS, much of which relates to adequate medical information, cytomorphology and dysplastic assessment and new molecular genetic information about these neoplasms. The revised WHO classification is the more accurate classification introduces refinements in morphologic interpretation and cytopenia assessment and addresses the influence of genetic information in MDS diagnosis and classification of patients and will allow for better guidance of treatment.

The evaluation of cytogenetic results is important for the classification and determination of the prognosis according to the revised International Prognostic Scoring System (IPSS-R). Immunophenotyping and molecular analysis will provide valuable information on diagnosis and prognosis.

Author details

Gamal Abdul Hamid[1*], Abdul Wahab Al-Nehmi[2] and Safa Shukry[1]

1 Faculty of Medicine and Health Sciences, University of Aden, Yemen

2 National Oncology Center, Sana'a, Yemen

*Address all correspondence to: drgamal2000@yahoo.com

References

[1] Jaffe ES, Harris NL, Stein H, et al. World Health Organization classification of tumours: Pathology and genetics of tumours of haematopoietic and lymphoid tissues. Annals of Oncology. 2002;**13**(3):490-491. DOI: 10.1093/annonc/mdf146

[2] Malcovati L, Germing U, Kuendgen A, et al. Time dependent prognostic scoring system for predicting survival and leukemic evolution in the myelodysplastic syndromes. Journal of Clinical Oncology. 2007;**25**:3503-3510. DOI: 10.1200/JCO.2006.08.5696

[3] Rollison DE, Howlader N, Smith MT, et al. Epidemiology of myelodysplastic syndromes and chronic myeloproliferative disorders in the United States, 2001-2004, using data from the NAACCR and SEER programs. Blood. 2008;**112**:45-52. DOI: 10.1182/blood-2008-01-134858

[4] Lee JH, Shin YR, et al. Application of different prognostic scoring systems and comparison of the FAB and WHO classifications in Korean patients with myelodysplastic syndrome. Leukemia. 2003;**17**(2):305-313. DOI: 10.1038/sj.leu.2402798

[5] Arber DA, Orazi A, Hasserjian R, et al. The 2016 revision on the World Health Organization classification of myeloid neoplasms and acute leukemia. Blood. 2016;**127**:2391-2405. DOI: 10.1182/blood-2016-03-643544

[6] Greenberg PL, Tuechler H, Schanz J, et al. Cytopenia levels for aiding establishment of the diagnosis of myelodysplastic syndromes. Blood. 2016;**128**:2096-2097. DOI: 10.1182/blood-2016-07-728766

[7] National Comperhensive Cancer Network (NCCN). NCCN Clinical Practice Guidelines in Oncology (NCCN) Guideline. Myelodysplastic Syndrome Version 2.2017. 2017. Available from: http://www.jnccn.org/content/15/1/60.full.pdf+html

[8] Valent P, Horny HP, Bennet JM, et al. Definitions and standards in the diagnosis and treatment of the myelodysplastic syndromes: Consensus statements and report from a working conference. Leukemia Research. 2007;**31**:727-736. DOI: 10.1016/j.leukres.2006.11.009

[9] Bain BJ. Diagnostic from the blood smear. The New England Journal of Medicine. 2005;**353**:498-507. DOI: 10.1056/NEJMra043442

[10] Greeberg PL, Attar E, Bennett JM, et al. Myelodysplastic syndromes. Clinical practice Guideline in Oncology. Journal of the National Comprehensive Cancer Network. 2013;**11**(7):838-874. DOI: 10.6004/jnccn.2013.0104

[11] Vallesp T, Michele I, Cristina M, et al. Diagnosis, classification, and cytogenetic of myelodysplastic syndrome. Hematologica. 1998;**83**: 258-275. PubMed 9573680

[12] Mufti GJ, Bennett JM, Goasguen J, et al. Diagnosis and classification of myelodysplastic syndrome: International Working Group on Morphology of myelodysplastic syndrome (IWGM-MDS) consensus proposals for the definition and enumeration of myeloblasts and ring sideroblasts. Haematologica. 2008;**93**(11):1712-1717. DOI: 10.3324/haematol.13405

[13] Goasguen JE, Bennett J, Cox C, et al. Prognostic implication and characterization of the blast cell population in the myelodysplastic syndrome. Leukemia Research. 1991;**15**:1159-1165. DOI: 10.1016/0145-2126(91)90185-V

[14] Shukry S. Bone marrow examination in pancytopenic patients

[thesis]. Faculty of Medicine & Health Science, Aden University; 2006

[15] Abdul Hamid G, Shukry S. Patterns of pancytopenia in Yemen. Turkish Journal of Hematology. 2008;**25**:71-74. PMID: 27264442

[16] Greenberg PL, Stone RM, Al-Kali A, et al. Myelodysplastic syndromes, version 2.2017, NCCN clinical practice guidelines in oncology. Journal of the National Comprehensive Cancer Network. 2017;**15**:60-87. DOI: 10.6004/jnccn.2017.0007

[17] Goasguen JE, Bennett JM, Bain BJ, et al. Morphological evaluation of monocytes and their precursors. Haematologica. 2009;**94**:994-997. DOI: 10.3324/haematol.2008.005421

[18] Bennett JM, Catovsky D, Daniel MT, et al. Proposals for the classification of the myelodysplastic syndromes. British Journal of Haematology. 1982;**51**: 189-199. PMID: 6952920

[19] Schanz J, Tuechler H, Sole F, et al. New comprehensive cytogenetic scoring system for primary myelodysplastic syndrome (MDS) and oligoblastic acute leukemia after MDS, derived from an international database merge. Journal of Clinical Oncology. 2012;**30**(8):820-829. DOI: 10.1200/JCO.2011.35.6394

[20] Vardiman JW, Thiele J, Arber DA, et al. The 2008 revision of the World Health Organization (WHO) classification of myeloid neoplasms and acute leukemia: Rationale and important changes. Blood. 2009;**114**:937-951. DOI: 10.1182/blood-2009-03-209262

[21] Genovese G, Kahler AK, Handsaker RE, et al. Clonal hematopoiesis and blood cancer risk inferred from blood DNA sequence. The New England Journal of Medicine. 2014;**371**: 2477-2487. DOI: 10.1056/NEJMoa1409405

[22] Hong M, He G. The 2016 revision to the World Health Organization classification of myelodysplastic syndromes. Journal of Translational Internal Medicine. 2017;**5**(3):139-143. DOI: 10.1515/jtim-2017-0002

[23] Papaemmanuil E, Gerstung M, Malcovati L, et al. Clinical and biological implications of gene mutations in MDS [abstract]. Leukemia Research. 2013;**37**(Suppl 1):S9. DOI: 10.1182/blood-2013-08-518886

[24] Malcovati L, Karimi M, Papaemmanuil E, et al. SF3B1 mutation identifies a distinct subset of myelodysplastic syndrome with ring sideroblasts. Blood. 2015;**126**:233-241. DOI: 10.1182/blood-2015-03-633537

[25] Bejar R. Implications of molecular genetic diversity in MDS. Current Opinion in Hematology. 2017;**24**(2):73-78. DOI: 10.1097/MOH.0000000000000313

[26] Westers TM, Van der Velden VH, Alhan C, et al. Implementation of flow cytometry in the diagnostic work-up of myelodysplastic syndromes in a multicenter approach: Report from the Dutch working party on flow cytometry in MDS. Leukemia Research. 2012;**36**(4):422-430. DOI: 10.1016/j.leukres.2011.09.015

[27] Della Porta MG, Picone C. Diagnostic utility of flow cytometry in myelodysplastic syndromes. Mediterranean Journal of Hematology and Infectious Diseases. 2017;**9**(1):e2017017. DOI: 10.4084/MJHID.2017.017

[28] Van de Loosdrecht AA, Ireland R, Kern W, et al. Rationale for the clinical application of flow cytometry in patients with myelodysplastic syndromes: Position paper of an International Consortium and the European LeukemiaNet Working roup. Leukemia & Lymphoma. 2013;**54**(3):472-475. DOI: 10.3109/10428194.2012.718341

[29] Bennett JM. A comparative review of classification systems in myelodysplastic syndromes (MDS). Seminars in Oncology. 2005;**32** (4 Suppl 5):S3-S10. DOI: 10.1053/j.seminoncol.2005.06.021

[30] Tuzuner N, Cox C, Rowe JM, et al. Hypocellular myelodysplastic syndromes (MDS): New proposals. British Journal of Haematology. 1995;**91**:612-617. DOI: 10.1111/j.1365-2141.1995.tb05356.x

[31] Verhoef GEG, De Wolf-Peeters C, Ferrant A, et al. Myelodysplastic syndromes with bone marrow fibrosis: A myelodysplastic disorder with proliferative features. Annals of Hematology. 1991;**63**(5):235-241. DOI: 10.1007/BF01698371

[32] Harris NL, Jaffe ES, Diebold J, et al. World Health Organization of neoplastic diseases of the hematopoietic and lymphoid tissues: Report of the clinical advisory committee meeting—Airlie House, Virginia, November 1997. Journal of Clinical Oncology. 1999;**17**:3835-3849. DOI: 10.1200/JCO.1999.17.12.3835

[33] Cazzola M. Introduction to a review series: The 2016 revision of the WHO classification of tumors of hematopoietic and lymphoid tissues. Blood. 2016;**127**:2361-2364. DOI: 10.1182/blood-2016-03-657379

[34] Campo E, Swerdlow SH, Harris NL, et al. The 2008 WHO classification of lymphoid neoplasms and beyond: Evolving concepts and practical applications. Blood. 2011;**117**(19):5019-5032. DOI: 10.1182/blood-2011-01-293050

[35] Pellagatti A, Boultwood J. The molecular pathogenesis of the myelodysplastic syndromes. European Journal of Haematology. 2015;**95**(1): 3-15. DOI: 10.1111/ejh.12515

[36] Sanz GF. A lot to learn about allogeneic hematopoietic cell transplantation for chronic myelomonocytic. Biology of Blood and Marrow Transplantation. 2017;**23**(5):713-714. DOI: 10.1016/j.bbmt.2017.03.011

[37] Murthy GSG, Dhakal I, Mehta P. Incidence and survival outcomes of chronic myelomonocytic leukemia in the United States. Leukemia & Lymphoma. 2017;**58**(7):1648-1654. DOI: 10.1080/10428194.2016.1258700

[38] Hyjek E, Vardiman JW. Myelodysplastic/myeloproliferative neoplasms. Seminars in Diagnostic Pathology. 2011;**28**:283-297. DOI: 10.1053/j.semdp.2011.07.002

[39] Schuler E, Shroder M, Neukirchen I, et al. Refined medullary blast and white blood cell count based classification of chronic myelomonocytic leukemia. Leukemia Research. 2014;**38**(12):1413-1419. DOI: 10.1016/j.leukres.2014.09.00

[40] Selimoglu-Buet D, Wagner-Ballon O, Saada V, et al. Characteristic repartition of monocyte subsets as a diagnostic signature of chronic myelomonocytic leukemia. Blood. 2015;**125**(23):3618-3626. DOI: 10.1182/blood-2015-01-620781

[41] Ziegler-Heitbrock L, Ancuta P, Crowes S, et al. Nomenclature of monocytes and dendretic cells in blood. Blood. 2010;**116**(16):e74-e80. DOI: 10.1182/blood-2010-02-258558

[42] Bioochi L, Espinal Witter R, Geyer JT, et al. Development of monocytosis in patients with primary myelofibrosis indicates on accelerated phase of the disease. Modern Pathology. 2013;**26**(2):204-212. DOI: 10.1038/modpathol.2012.165

[43] Such E, Cervera J, Costa D, et al. Cytogenetic risk stratification in chronic myelomonocytic leukemia. Haematologica. 2011;**96**(3):375-383. DOI: 10.3324/haematol.2010.030957

Chapter 3

Myelodysplastic Syndrome and Autoimmune Disorders: Causal Relationship or Coincidence?

Kam A. Newman, Mojtaba Akhtari and Sheda Heidarian

Abstract

Myelodysplastic syndromes are heterogeneous group of clonal hematologic malignancies characterized by peripheral blood cytopenias secondary to the ineffective hematopoiesis. ADs are frequently reported in MDS, the incidence ranging from 10 to 30%, and particularly ADs are more frequently seen at CMML. ADs may prone patient to MDS, especially when immune suppressors such as azathioprine are used for the underlying AD. Both innate and adaptive immune systems, and different cytokines including interleukins, TNF-α, and C-X-C motif chemokine 10 (CXCL10) contribute in immune dysregulation of MDS. Vasculitis, seronegative rheumatoid arthritis, SLE, Behçet's disease, RP, and AIHA are just some of the ADs occurring concomitantly with MDS. Although hematopoietic growth factors are recommended by the American Society of Clinical Oncology (ASCO), it has been recognized from several case reports that treatment of the underlying MDS may resolve the associated autoimmune disorders. The heterogeneity and complexity of pathology, clinical manifestations, response to therapy, and prognosis of MDS and its immune dysregulation make the prognosis of MDS with autoimmune diseases a matter of debate. Better understanding of the immune dysregulation of MDS in the molecular level may help to design prospective, double blind clinical trials to find the best treatment options for autoimmune disorders associated with MDS.

Keywords: autoimmune disorders (ADs), myelodysplastic syndrome (MDS), chronic myelomonocytic leukemia (CMML), Behçet's disease, systemic lupus erythematosus (SLE), azathioprine, azacitidine, tumor necrosis factor alpha (TNF-α), regulatory T-cells (Treg), autoimmune hemolytic anemia (AIHA), vasculitis, chronic inflammatory demyelinating polyneuropathy (CIDP), neutrophilic dermatosis, Henoch-Schonlein purpura, relapsing polychondritis (RP), granulomatosis with polyangiitis (GPA), giant cell arteritis (GCA), polyarteritis nodosa (PAN)

1. Introduction

Myelodysplastic syndromes (MDS) are characterized by peripheral blood cytopenias secondary to the ineffective hematopoiesis, and represent a heterogeneous group of clonal hematologic malignancies in which abnormal multipotent progenitor cells are involved. As a result, there is an increased risk of bleeding diathesis and anemia requiring frequent transfusions, infections, and progression to acute myeloid leukemia [1–4]. It is a very well-known fact that a large spectrum of genetic mutations is involved in MDS pathogenesis that may affect clinical outcome and response to the treatment. These genetic mutations may control cell cycle by affecting key proteins of spliceosome, DNA repair, kinase signaling, tumor suppressor genes, and transcription factors, changing bone marrow micro environment, resulting in hypercellular bone marrow with peripheral cytopenias through enhanced programmed cell death (PCD) and bone marrow dysfunction [5, 6]. To overcome programmed cell death, hematopoietic growth factors such as erythropoiesis stimulating agents (ESAs) and granulocyte colony stimulating factor (G-CSF) are the 1st step in management of the low-grade MDS recommended by the American Society of Clinical Oncology (ASCO) to reduce early apoptosis [1].

Thrombopoietic stimulating agents (TSAs), ESAs, G-CSF, antithymocyte globulin (ATG) [7], lenalidomide [8], and hypomethylating agents are some of the non-transplantation options for management of the MDS patients suggesting that immune dysregulation plays a pivotal role in MDS pathogenesis [1]. Although its etiology is not clear, it has been shown that natural killer (NK) cell activity and its response to chemokines is decreased in MDS, and natural killer cells will be progressively more dysfunctional with MDS progression [9]. It has been shown that although dysfunctional regulatory T-cells (Treg), cells in charge of suppressing T helper (Th) activity, contribute in early stages of MDS, Th expands in the later stages of MDS, and there function is significantly reduced with treatment [10].

Tumor necrosis factor alpha (TNF-α) level is higher in bone marrow and peripheral blood plasma of MDS patients, and may reflect an unfavorable outcome [11, 12]. Study shows that plasma level of 19 cytokines are significantly altered compared with normal individuals, among all of them, C-X-C motif chemokine 10 (CXCL10) and interleukin 6 were associated with shortened survival [13]. The relationship between shorter survival and interleukin 6 levels is very well known, and high producing genotypes of both TNF-α and interleukin 6 are highly associated with transfusion dependency for both anemia and thrombocytopenia, and severity of the bicytopenias [14]. Interferon regulatory factor-1 (IRF-1), a transcriptional activator of interferon system, has anti oncogenic properties, inhibits tumor formation, and regulates innate immune response. It has been shown that IRF-1 mRNA is 10 fold decreased in MDS patients, while it is increased in MDS patients with autoimmune disorders, showing that IRF-1 may promote inflammation and autoimmunity and has a protective roll in MDS patient's [15].

Although it has been reported that MDS is significantly associated with autoimmune disorders, it may occur secondary to the autoimmune disorders per se [16] or exposure to the therapeutic agents used for treatment of autoimmune disorders. A retrospective study in Sweden on 1662 MDS patients and 42,878 matched controls revealed that underlying autoimmune disorder increased risk of MDS by 2.1 with highest risks observed with prior autoimmune hemolytic anemia (AIHA), polyarteritis nodosa (PAN), granulomatosis with polyangiitis (GPA), giant cell arteritis (GCA) and aplastic anemia. It was speculated that chronic stimulation of the immune system may act as a trigger and prone the patient to MDS [17]. In a retrospective study of 2471 patients, it was found that MDS occurred subsequent to autoimmune disorders, most commonly rheumatoid arthritis, Sjogren's syndrome, systemic lupus erythematosus, polyarteritis nodosa, discoid lupus erythematosus, and pernicious anemia were associated with MDS [18]. In a case control study of 80 for MDS patients, it was found that there is strong and statistically significant evidence that MDS occurred after autoimmune disorders with Grave's disease and Hashimoto's thyroiditis were among the most important disorders [19]. There is a case report of limited granulomatosis with polyangiitis (GPA) treated with corticosteroids, who did develop myelodysplastic syndrome, papillary thyroid carcinoma, and gastric adenocarcinoma [20].

There are several reports regarding therapy related MDS in population with autoimmune disorders who underwent disease modifying antirheumatic drugs (DMARDs) therapy. In a retrospective case-control study of 40,011 patients with 27 kinds of autoimmune disorders, 311 patients met the inclusion criteria, 86 of them had MDS, and found azathioprine exposure has increased 7 fold myeloid neoplasms in a median of 8 years. In this study, methotrexate, and mycophenolate mofetil did not elevate the risk of myeloid neoplasms [21]. However, there is a case report regarding association of low-dose oral methotrexate therapy with MDS in a rheumatoid arthritis patient [22]. In another study, from 370 rheumatologic patients who received azathioprine for at least 1 year, 59 patients underwent bone marrow examination and 2 of them found to have MDS. This study revealed that risk of secondary MDS is 100 fold higher in patients who received azathioprine for their rheumatologic disorders. Chromosomal examination of the patients with MDS secondary to the azathioprine showed abnormalities of chromosome 7 in majority of them (8 out of 10) [23]. There is also evidence that MDS patients who have autoimmune disorders might respond to hypomethylating agents such as azacitidine and decitabine [24].

2. Rheumatologic manifestations of MDS

It is a very well-known fact that about 10–30% of MDS patients may present with a variety of autoimmune or laboratory manifestations or develop an autoimmune disorder. These manifestations are polymorphic and include leukocytoclastic vasculitis, clubbing, peripheral neuropathy, autoimmune hemolytic anemia, polyarthritis, myositis, acute or systemic vasculitis, Raynaud's phenomenon, polyarteritis nodosa, vitiligo, iritis, colonic ulcerations, pulmonary involvement, and reported autoimmune disorders include rheumatoid arthritis, Sjogren's disease, giant cell arteritis, polymyalgia rheumatica, relapsing polychondritis, Behçet's disease, and systemic lupus erythematosus. Although autoimmune manifestations are mostly seen during the course of MDS, autoimmune disorders may occur before MDS diagnosis. Laboratory manifestations of MDS include hypergammaglobulinemia, hypogammaglobulinemia, monoclonal gammopathy, positive direct antiglobulin test (DAT), positive ANA, rheumatoid factor, cryoglobulinemia, and anti-double-stranded DNA.

3. Autoimmune disorders in myelodysplastic syndrome

Several studies support that autoimmune disorders may occur in the setting of MDS, and treating MDS with immunosuppressors may improve the autoimmune disorder. Although there were several case reports of MDS preceding autoimmune disorders, the first comprehensive retrospective study in 1986 on 104 MDS patients revealed two patients had pernicious anemia, two had hypothyroidism, and one had both pernicious anemia and hypothyroidism [23]. Later, in a retrospective study in 1994, five patients with MDS reviewed and revealed polyarthritis with positive rheumatoid factor (RF) and necrotizing vasculitis [25]. In another retrospective study in 1995, 221 patients with MDS reviewed and found 30 patients with autoimmune disorders, and categorized patient to three categories of acute systemic vasculitis or autoimmune disorder, chronic or isolated autoimmune phenomena, and classic connective tissue disorders. Skin vasculitis, arthritis, and fever were among the most common autoimmune manifestations [26].

A case series in 2002 showed various autoimmune paraneoplastic disorders including vasculitis, pyoderma gangrenosum, Coombs negative autoimmune hemolytic anemia, autoimmune thrombocytopenia, and chronic inflammatory demyelinating polyneuropathy (CIDP) with good response to immunosuppressive therapy [27]. In a retrospective review of 235 MDS patients autoimmune manifestations such as skin vasculitis (24%), noninfectious fever (13%), arthralgia and arthritis (13%), peripheral neuropathy (10%), and pulmonary infiltrates (8%) were more common than systemic vasculitis [28]. In a cohort of 1408 patients with MDS, 391 (28%) had autoimmune disorders, with hypothyroidism (44%), as the most prevalent, and idiopathic thrombocytopenic purpura (12%), rheumatoid arthritis (10%), and psoriasis (7%) were among the common manifestations of autoimmune diseases [29].

In a retrospective study of 67 MDS patients with autoimmune diseases, neutrophilic dermatosis was the most common autoimmune disease (35.8%), followed by Behçet's disease (14.9%), and rheumatoid arthritis (13.4%) [30].

3.1 Vasculitis

The association between MDS and vasculitis is rare, but more common than solid tumors, and has been described for decades. Cutaneous vasculitis presents by palpable purpura mainly in lower extremities that involves small vessels and is characterized by perivascular inflammation and vessel wall damage by infiltrating neutrophils. Although both cutaneous and systemic vasculitis has been reported in MDS patients, at times they can be seen together in MDS patients. For instance, in a case series of 6 biopsy proven cutaneous vasculitis patients with MDS, 3 patients had evidence of systemic vasculitis [31]. In one case, MDS patient with biopsy proven cutaneous vasculitis developed acute myeloid leukemia within 4 months of vasculitis diagnosis [32]. Henoch-Schonlein purpura, a small vessel vasculitis with IgA dominant immune deposits has been described in MDS patients [33].

The association of MDS and polyarteritis nodosa (PAN) type medium-vessel vasculitis has been reported [34]. In a retrospective study of 8 patients with chronic myelomonocytic leukemia (CMML), with vasculitis involved the medium-vessel, fulfilling the criteria for classic PAN, the presentation was non-specific, and patients developed atypical manifestations [35]. There is a case report of 43-year-old man who qualified for a diagnosis of PAN and developed systemic vasculitis at the time of chronic myelomonocytic leukemia (CMML) diagnosis [36]. There is a report of two cases with CMML who presented with PAN-like systemic vasculitis with bilateral perirenal hemorrhage and negative antineutrophil cytoplasmic antibody with improvement of vasculitis with systemic steroids [37].

Although most MDS associated vasculitis described as leukocytoclastic vasculitis, published case reports documented large vessel vasculitis as autoimmune complication of MDS. Aortitis has been reported as an autoimmune manifestation of an MDS patient at presentation [38]. There is a report of two MDS cases that presented with acute large vessel vasculitis with rapid improvement with systemic steroids [39]. In a retrospective analysis of 271 temporal arteritis patients, it was found that 20 patients had malignancy, of which 11 patients had MDS, favoring a relationship between large vessel vasculitis and MDS [40]. There is a case report of Takayasu's arteritis diagnosed shortly after diagnosis of MDS, with progression to AML regardless of improvement of vasculitis with immunosuppressive treatment [41]. There is a case report of a 71-year-old woman presenting with fever, neck pain, anemia, and thrombocytopenia, with positive positron emission tomography (PET)/CT scan of the aorta and carotid arteries with negative temporal artery biopsy who received the diagnosis of MDS after a bone marrow aspiration analysis [42, 43].

3.2 Behçet's disease

A multisystem, chronic inflammatory disease of unknown etiology, Behçet's disease (BD) is characterized by recurrent oral and genital ulcers, uveitis, arthritis, and vascular involvement of several organs including pulmonary, central nervous system and gastrointestinal tract. In a retrospective study of 805 BD patients, 16 patients had MDS, from which 43.8% had BD prior to MDS, 18.7% diagnosed after MDS and 37.5% had concurrent BD and MDS. It has been shown that trisomy 8 has been accumulated in all of BD patients with MDS, and these patients more likely to be female, older age, and have fever and ileocecal ulcerations [44]. In a retrospective study of 46 MDS patients, 8 patients had trisomy 8, 5 of them had multiple intestinal ulcers, a common feature of BD. Two of the MDS patients with trisomy 8 and multiple intestinal ulcers were treated with granulocyte-colony stimulating factor (G-CSF), aggravating their symptoms, suggesting G-CSF should be used cautiously in this subgroup of MDS patients [45]. There is several case reports of BD associated with MDS [46–49]. In a case report of two patients with BD and MDS, it has been suggested that PET/CT may help diagnosis of both BD and MDS with high uptake by bone marrow in MDS patients and genital and gastrointestinal aphthous ulcers in BD patients [50]. It has been suggested that the frequency of gastrointestinal involvement is more common in MDS-associated BD patients than general BD population [51].

3.3 Inflammatory arthritis

There are several case reports and small series of inflammatory arthritis and MDS co-occurrence. In a retrospective study of 28 MDS patients, 8 had acute seronegative inflammatory arthritis with good response of arthritis to steroids [52]. In a French multicenter retrospective study of 22 patients with MDS, 77% of patients had polyarthritis, and 68% had symmetric joint involvement. Radiologic erosions are rare, and MDS associated arthritis is more frequent in refractory anemia with excess blast (RAEB) [53].

3.4 Miscellaneous

There are several case reports of relapsing polychondritis (RP) presenting as a paraneoplastic disorder in the setting of MDS [54, 55]. In a retrospective study of hematological changes in 19 patients with relapsing polychondritis, MDS was found in three RP patients [56]. Autoimmune hemolytic anemia has been reported in association with MDS [57–59]. Association of systemic lupus erythematosus and MDS has been reported [60–62].

3.5 Immunological abnormalities

It is a very well-known fact that a spectrum of immunological abnormalities occur in MDS. In a retrospective study of 104 MDS patients, 12.5% had monoclonal gammopathy, 19% had low immunoglobulin levels, 32% had polyclonal rise in serum immunoglobulin level, and 8.1% had positive direct antiglobulin test (DAT) [25]. In a case series of 142 patients with MDS and CMML, 23.2% had non-organ specific autoantibody ANA as the most frequent serologic finding [25]. Thrombocytopenia is a common finding in MDS, and can be seen in up to two third of the patients. In a study of 54 MDS patients with no treatment of transfusions, direct platelet immunofluorescence test for platelet associated IgG was positive in 28 patients. Patients with higher amount of platelet associated IgG, had significantly higher mean platelet volume (MPV), thrombocytopenia and worse outcome [63].

4. Prognosis

It has been suggested that appearance of skin vasculitis in MDS patients may reflect acute myeloid leukemia transformation. In a prospective study of 157 MDS patients for a median of 44 months, 15 patients (9.55%) experienced skin lesions, and neutrophilic dermatosis (7, 4.46%), specific lesions (5, 3.18%), cutaneous vasculitis (2, 1.27%) and Behçet's disease (1, 0.63%) were reported. This study revealed that neutrophilic dermatosis was more prevalent in MDS patients, may confer the higher risk of acute myeloid leukemia transformation [64]. In another study of 84 newly diagnosed MDS patients, correlation of cutaneous findings with immunologic parameters and prognostic features of MDS examined, and revealed that 21 patients had skin lesions at presentation, and skin manifestations were a significant predictor of the high-risk MDS subgroup [65].

In a retrospective study of 153 MDS patients, 12% had autoimmune diseases, and 63% has at least one immunological abnormality in test results. In this study, the survival of patients without autoimmune diseases was better than patients with autoimmune disease [66]. However, in a 4 year prospective study of 70 MDS patients, 53 patients without and 13 patients with autoimmune disease, there was no particular difference concerning prognosis between two groups. And patients with autoimmune diseases were not statistically different in survival compared with MDS patients without autoimmune disease [67].

5. Treatment

Autoimmune disorders associated with MDS may predate or occur after MDS diagnosis, and their treatment many be associated with significant side effects in MDS patients. It has been recognized from several case reports that treatment of the underlying MDS may resolve the associated autoimmune disorders. In a transfusion dependent MDS patient who was receiving G-CSF and erythropoietin, neutrophilic dermatosis did not improve with G-CSF withholding. Two months after starting 5-azacitidine, a hypomethylating agent, the skin rash completely resolved, and did not recur after 2 years [68]. In another case series of 3 MDS patients with autoimmune disorders, 5-azacitidine improved both MDS and autoimmune disorders although long term steroid could not be tapered [69].

In a retrospective study of 123 MDS patients with autoimmune disorders, 118 patients (96%) were treated with steroids, and 48% of patients were required a second line treatment for refractory disease or relapse. Although autoimmune disorder treatment did not improve MDS, MDS treatment with 5-azacitidine improved the autoimmune disorder in 9 out of 11 (80%) of patients [70]. In another retrospective study of 123 MDS/CMML patients with autoimmune disorders, 28 patients received at least 5 cycles of azacitidine, 20 of them did not respond to steroids. In 86% of MDS/CMML patients, clinical autoimmune syndromes improved by azacitidine, and prednisone dose tapered in 64% of patients [71].

The overall effect of biologic medications efficacy in MDS patients who presented with autoimmune disorder is not clear. As of today, there is only one retrospective study of MDS patients with autoimmune disorders and biologic medications. In this study of at least one biologic medication, 29 patients followed for at least 3 years. 89% of patients received a biologic after failure or intolerance of two disease modifying anti rheumatic agents (DMARDs), however, 11% of patients received biologics as a first line treatment. Except rituximab, a CD-20 blocker, mainly for vasculitis (58% response), there was partial or insufficient response to

TNF-α antagonists, and their efficacy is much less in autoimmune disorders associated with MDS than autoimmune disorders without MDS. Overall, response rate to 5-azacitidine in MDS-associated autoimmune disorders was 67% in favor of a causality relationship between MDS and autoimmune disorders [72].

6. Conclusion

Myelodysplastic syndromes are a heterogeneous group of progressive clonal hematopoietic stem cell disorders characterized by a varying degree of peripheral cytopenia, and increased probability of transformation to acute myeloid leukemia. MDS and particularly CMML are frequently associated with a variety of autoimmune disorders that can be diagnosed concomitantly with MDS or before or after MDS. The heterogeneity and complexity of pathology, clinical manifestations, response to therapy, and prognosis of MDS and its immune dysregulation makes the prognosis of MDS with autoimmune diseases a matter of debate. Prospective, randomized studies are required to confirm the autoimmune diseases role in MDS prognosis.

Acknowledgements

The authors would like to thank Mr. Dixon Bennet for his technical assistance.

Disclosure

None.

Author details

Kam A. Newman[1]*, Mojtaba Akhtari[2] and Sheda Heidarian[3]

1 Eisenhower Rheumatology Specialty Clinic, Eisenhower Health, Internal Medicine Residency Program, Mike and Jan Salta Health Center, Rancho Mirage, CA, United States

2 Clinical Medicine, Jane Anne Nohl Division of Hematology and Center for the Study of Blood Diseases, USC/Norris Cancer Center, Los Angeles, CA, United States

3 President Elect, Medical Staff, Eisenhower Health, Rancho Mirage, CA, United States

*Address all correspondence to: knewman@eisenhowerhealth.org

References

[1] Newman K, Maness-Harris L, El-Hemaidi I, Akhtari M. Revisiting use of growth factors in myelodysplastic syndromes. Asian Pacific Journal of Cancer Prevention. 2012;**13**(4): 1081-1091

[2] Sallman DA, Tanaka TN, List A, Bejar R. SOHO state of the art update and next questions: Biology and treatment of myelodysplastic syndromes. Clinical Lymphoma, Myeloma & Leukemia. 2017;**17**(10): 613-620

[3] Hidalgo-López JE, Kanagal-Shamanna R, Quesada AE, Thakral B, Hu Z, Mitsuhashi T, et al. Progress in myelodysplastic syndromes: Clinicopathologic correlations and immune checkpoints. Clinical Lymphoma, Myeloma & Leukemia. 2017;**17S**:S16-S25

[4] Akhtrai M. When to treat myelodysplastic syndrome. Oncology (Williston Park, N.Y.). 2011;**25**(6): 480-486

[5] Raza A, Mundle S, Iftikhar A, Gregory S, Marcus B, Khan Z, et al. Simultaneous assessment of cell kinetics and programmed cell death in bone marrow biopsies of myelodysplastics reveals extensive apoptosis as the probable basis for ineffective hematopoiesis. American Journal of Hematology. 1995;**48**(3):143-154

[6] Shallis RM, Ahmad R, Zeidan AM. The genetic and molecular pathogenesis of myelodysplastic syndromes. European Journal of Haematology. 2018. DOI: 10.1111/ejh.13092 [Epub ahead of print]

[7] Molldrem JJ, Caples M, Mavroudis D, Plante M, Young NS, Barrett AJ. Antithymocyte globulin for patients with myelodysplastic syndrome. British Journal of Haematology. 1997;**99**(3): 699-705

[8] List A, Dewald G, Bennett J, Giagounidis A, Raza A, Feldman E, et al. Lenalidomide in the myelodysplastic syndrome with chromosome 5q deletion. The New England Journal of Medicine. 2006;**355**(14):1456-1465

[9] Kiladjian JJ, Bourgeois E, Lobe I, Braun T, Visentin G, Bourhis JH, et al. Cytolytic function and survival of natural killer cells are severely altered in myelodysplastic syndromes. Leukemia. 2006;**20**(3):463-470

[10] Kotsianidis I, Bouchliou I, Nakou E, Spanoudakis E, Margaritis D, Christophoridou AV, et al. Kinetics, function and bone marrow trafficking of CD4+CD25+FOXP3+ regulatory T cells in myelodysplastic syndromes (MDS). Leukemia. 2009;**23**(3):510-518

[11] Stifter G, Heiss S, Gastl G, Tzankov A, Stauder R. Over-expression of tumor necrosis factor-alpha in bone marrow biopsies from patients with myelodysplastic syndromes: Relationship to anemia and prognosis. European Journal of Haematology. 2005;**75**(6):485-491

[12] Tsimberidou AM, Estey E, Wen S, Pierce S, Kantarjian H, Albitar M, et al. The prognostic significance of cytokine levels in newly diagnosed acute myeloid leukemia and high-risk myelodysplastic syndromes. Cancer. 2008;**113**(7): 1605-1613

[13] Pardanani A, Finke C, Lasho TL, Al-Kali A, Begna KH, Hanson CA, et al. IPSS-independent prognostic value of plasma CXCL10, IL-7 and IL-6 levels in myelodysplastic syndromes. Leukemia. 2012;**26**(4):693-699

[14] Bestach Y, Nagore VP, Flores MG, González J, Arbelbide J, Watman N, et al. Influence of TNF and IL6 gene polymorphisms on the severity of

cytopenias in argentine patients with myelodysplastic syndromes. Annals of Hematology. 2017;**96**(8):1287-1295

[15] Giannouli S, Tzoanopoulos D, Ritis K, Kartalis G, Moutsopoulos HM, Voulgarelis M. Autoimmune manifestations in human myelodysplasia: A positive correlation with interferon regulatory factor-1 (IRF-1) expression. Annals of the Rheumatic Diseases. 2004;**63**(5):578-582

[16] Wilson AB, Neogi T, Prout M, Jick S. Relative risk of myelodysplastic syndromes in patients with autoimmune disorders in the General Practice Research Database. Cancer Epidemiology. 2014;**38**(5):544-549

[17] Kristinsson SY, Björkholm M, Hultcrantz M, Derolf ÅR, Landgren O, Goldin LR. Chronic immune stimulation might act as a trigger for the development of acute myeloid leukemia or myelodysplastic syndromes. Journal of Clinical Oncology. 2011;**29**(21):2897-2903

[18] Anderson LA, Pfeiffer RM, Landgren O, Gadalla S, Berndt SI, Engels EA. Risks of myeloid malignancies in patients with autoimmune conditions. British Journal of Cancer. 2009;**100**(5):822-828

[19] Dalamaga M, Petridou E, Cook FE, Trichopoulos D. Risk factors for myelodysplastic syndromes: A case-control study in Greece. Cancer Causes & Control. 2002;**13**(7):603-608

[20] Cheon YH, Kim MG, Kim JE, Ha CY, Lee SI, Kim HO. Multiple malignancies in a patient with limited granulomatosis with polyangiitis without immunosuppressive therapy. Modern Rheumatology. 2016;**26**(3):450-453

[21] Ertz-Archambault N, Kosiorek H, Taylor GE, Kelemen K, Dueck A, Castro J, et al. Association of therapy for autoimmune disease with myelodysplastic syndromes and acute myeloid leukemia. JAMA Oncology. 2017;**3**(7):936-943

[22] Okamoto H, Teramura M, Kamatani N. Myelodysplastic syndrome associated with low-dose methotrexate in rheumatoid arthritis. The Annals of Pharmacotherapy. 2004;**38**(1):172-173

[23] Knipp S, Hildebrandt B, Richter J, Haas R, Germing U, Gattermann N. Secondary myelodysplastic syndromes following treatment with azathioprine are associated with aberrations of chromosome 7. Haematologica. 2005;**90**(5):691-693

[24] Al Ustwani O, Ford LA, Sait SJ, Block AM, Barcos M, Vigil CE, et al. Myelodysplastic syndromes and autoimmune diseases—Case series and review of literature. Leukemia Research. 2013;**37**(8):894-899

[25] Mufti GJ, Figes A, Hamblin TJ, Oscier DG, Copplestone JA. Immunological abnormalities in myelodysplastic syndromes. I. Serum immunoglobulins and autoantibodies. British Journal of Haematology. 1986;**63**(1):143-147

[26] Kuzmich PV, Ecker GA, Karsh J. Rheumatic manifestations in patients with myelodysplastic and myeloproliferative diseases. The Journal of Rheumatology. 1994;**21**(9):1649-1654

[27] Enright H, Jacob HS, Vercellotti G, Howe R, Belzer M, Miller W. Paraneoplastic autoimmune phenomena in patients with myelodysplastic syndromes: Response to immunosuppressive therapy. British Journal of Haematology. 1995;**91**(2):403-408

[28] Saif MW, Hopkins JL, Gore SD. Autoimmune phenomena in patients with myelodysplastic syndromes and

chronic myelomonocytic leukemia. Leukemia & Lymphoma. 2002;**43**(11): 2083-2092

[29] de Hollanda A, Beucher A, Henrion D, Ghali A, Lavigne C, Lévesque H, et al. Systemic and immune manifestations in myelodysplasia: A multicenter retrospective study. Arthritis Care & Research (Hoboken). 2011;**63**(8):1188-1194

[30] Komrokji RS, Kulasekararaj A, Al Ali NH, Kordasti S, Bart-Smith E, Craig BM, et al. Autoimmune diseases and myelodysplastic syndromes. American Journal of Hematology. 2016;**91**(5): E280-E283

[31] Lee SJ, Park JK, Lee EY, Joo SH, Jung KC, Lee EB, et al. Certain autoimmune manifestations are associated with distinctive karyotypes and outcomes in patients with myelodysplastic syndrome: A retrospective cohort study. Medicine (Baltimore). 2016;**95**(13): e3091

[32] Green AR, Shuttleworth D, Bowen DT, Bentley DP. Cutaneous vasculitis in patients with myelodysplasia. British Journal of Haematology. 1990;**74**(3): 364-365

[33] Pirayesh A, Verbunt RJ, Kluin PM, Meinders AE, De Meijer PH. Myelodysplastic syndrome with vasculitic manifestations. Journal of Internal Medicine. 1997;**242**(5):425-431

[34] Blanco R, Gonzalez-Gay MA, Ibañez D, Lopez-Viana A, Ferran C, Regueira A, et al. Henoch-Schönlein purpura as clinical presentation of a myelodysplastic syndrome. Clinical Rheumatology. 1997;**16**(6):626-628

[35] Brickner LA, Scannell KA. Medium-vessel PAN-type vasculitis associated with myelodysplastic syndrome and presenting as bilateral perinephric hematomas. Clinical and Experimental Rheumatology. 1997;**15**(2):221-222

[36] Hamidou MA, Boumalassa A, Larroche C, El Kouri D, Blétry O, Grolleau JY. Systemic medium-sized vessel vasculitis associated with chronic myelomonocytic leukemia. Seminars in Arthritis and Rheumatism. 2001;**31**(2): 119-126

[37] Oostvogels R, Petersen EJ, Chauffaille ML, Abrahams AC. Systemic vasculitis in myelodysplastic syndromes. The Netherlands Journal of Medicine. 2012;**70**(2):63-68

[38] Aslangul-Castier E, Papo T, Amoura Z, Baud O, Leblond V, Charlotte F, et al. Systemic vasculitis with bilateral perirenal haemorrhage in chronic myelomonocytic leukaemia. Annals of the Rheumatic Diseases. 2000;**59**(5): 390-393

[39] Lopez FF, Vaidyan PB, Mega AE, Schiffman FJ. Aortitis as a manifestation of myelodysplastic syndrome. Postgraduate Medical Journal. 2001; **77**(904):116-118

[40] Steurer M, Fritsche G, Tzankov A, Gotwald T, Sturm W, Konwalinka G, et al. Large-vessel arteritis and myelodysplastic syndrome: Report of two cases. European Journal of Haematology. 2004;**73**(2):128-133

[41] Liozon E, Loustaud V, Fauchais AL, Soria P, Ly K, Ouattara B, et al. Concurrent temporal (giant cell) arteritis and malignancy: Report of 20 patients with review of the literature. The Journal of Rheumatology. 2006; **33**(8):1606-1614

[42] Cohen MJ, Shyman A, Klein M, Ben-Yehuda A, Rubinow A, Or R, et al. Large vessel (Takayasu's) arteritis in a patient with myelodysplastic syndrome: Is there a common pathogenesis? Clinical Lymphoma, Myeloma & Leukemia. 2011;**11**(1):60-63

[43] Katsuyama T, Uchida HA, Toma K, Maeda Y, Hirota D, Umebayashi R, et al.

Large vessel vasculitis with myelodysplastic syndrome. Internal Medicine. 2014;**53**(1):63-66

[44] Shen Y, Ma HF, Luo D, Cai JF, Zou J, Guan JL. High incidence of gastrointestinal ulceration and cytogenetic aberration of trisomy 8 as typical features of Behçet's disease associated with myelodysplastic syndrome: A series of 16 consecutive Chinese patients from the shanghai Behçet's disease database and comparison with the literature. BioMed Research International. 2018;**2018**: 8535091

[45] Kimura S, Kuroda J, Akaogi T, Hayashi H, Kobayashi Y, Kondo M. Trisomy 8 involved in myelodysplastic syndromes as a risk factor for intestinal ulcers and thrombosis—Behçet's syndrome. Leukemia & Lymphoma. 2001;**42**(1–2):115-121

[46] Lee WS, Kang MH, Hwang JH, Oh YJ, Yoo WH. Allogeneic hematopoietic stem cell transplantation for refractory Behcet's disease with myelodysplastic syndrome: A case report. International Journal of Rheumatic Diseases. 2017; **20**(11):1860-1861

[47] Alekberova Z, Gorodetskiy V, Izmailova F, Radenska-Lopovok S, Talybova E, Evsikova M, et al. Behçet's disease and comorbidity: Internal case reports and literature review. Rheumatology International. 2015; **35**(10):1743-1747

[48] Takizawa Y, Setoguchi K, Kobayashi T, Kuwata G. Severe gastrointestinal disease development coinciding with the progression of myelodysplastic syndrome after a long-term mild course of Behcet's disease. International Journal of Rheumatic Diseases. 2017;**20**(11):1856-1859

[49] Kovacs E, Nemeth H, Telek B, Ujfalusi A, Balogh E, Pasztor E, et al. Behçet's disease in a patient with myelodysplastic syndrome. Clinical Lymphoma & Myeloma. 2009;**9**(6): 459-461

[50] Ito K, Kubota K. 18F-FDG PET/CT findings in two cases with myelodysplastic syndrome accompanied by Behçet's disease. Clinical Nuclear Medicine. 2016;**41**(8):e392-e393

[51] Esatoglu SN, Hatemi G, Salihoglu A, Hatemi I, Soysal T, Celik AF. A reappraisal of the association between Behçet's disease, myelodysplastic syndrome and the presence of trisomy 8: A systematic literature review. Clinical and Experimental Rheumatology. 2015; **33**(6 Supp. 94):S145-S151

[52] George SW, Newman ED. Seronegative inflammatory arthritis in the myelodysplastic syndromes. Seminars in Arthritis and Rheumatism. 1992;**21**(6):345-354

[53] Mekinian A, Braun T, Decaux O, Falgarone G, Toussirot E, Raffray L, et al. Inflammatory arthritis in patients with myelodysplastic syndromes: A multicenter retrospective study and literature review of 68 cases. Medicine (Baltimore). 2014;**93**(1):1-10

[54] Salahuddin N, Libman BS, Lunde JH, Kay J, Cooper SM. The association of relapsing polychondritis and myelodysplastic syndrome: Report of three cases. Journal of Clinical Rheumatology. 2000;**6**(3):146-149

[55] Van Besien K, Tricot G, Hoffman R. Relapsing polychondritis: A paraneoplastic syndrome associated with myelodysplastic syndromes. American Journal of Hematology. 1992; **40**(1):47-50

[56] Diebold L, Rauh G, Jäger K, Löhrs U. Bone marrow pathology in relapsing polychondritis: High frequency of myelodysplastic syndromes. British Journal of Haematology. 1995;**89**(4): 820-830

[57] Oren H, Uçar C, Gülen H, Duman M, Irken G. Autoimmune hemolytic anemia occurring with myelodysplastic syndrome: Report of a pediatric case and review of the literature. Annals of Hematology. 2001;**80**(9):540-542

[58] Lin JT, Wang WS, Yen CC, Chiou TJ, Liu JH, Hsiao LT, et al. Myelodysplastic syndrome complicated by autoimmune hemolytic anemia: Remission of refractory anemia following mycophenolate mofetil. Annals of Hematology. 2002;**81**(12): 723-726

[59] Sokol RJ, Hewitt S, Booker DJ. Erythrocyte autoantibodies, autoimmune haemolysis, and myelodysplastic syndromes. Journal of Clinical Pathology. 1989;**42**(10): 1088-1091

[60] Ng HS, Ng HW, Sinniah R, Feng PH. A case of systemic lupus erythematosus with sideroblastic anaemia terminating in erythroleukaemia. Annals of the Rheumatic Diseases. 1981;**40**(4): 422-426

[61] Jiménez-Balderas FJ, Morales-Polanco MR, Gutierrez L. Acute sideroblastic anemia in active systemic lupus erythematosus. Lupus. 1994;**3**(3): 157-159

[62] Montoro J, Gallur L, Merchán B, Molero A, Roldán E, Martínez-Valle F, Villacampa G, Navarrete M, Ortega M, Castellví J, Saumell S, Bobillo S, Bosch F, Valcárcel D. Autoimmune disorders are common in myelodysplastic syndrome patients and confer an adverse impact on outcomes. Ann Hematol. 2018;**97**(8): 1349-1356

[63] Gilli SC, de Souza Medina S, de Castro V, Fernandes LG, Saad ST. Platelet associated IgG may be related with thrombocytopenia in patients with myelodysplastic syndromes. Leukemia Research. 2012;**36**(5):554-559

[64] Farah C, Bulai Livideanu C, Jegu J, Paul C, Viraben R, Lamant L, et al. Prevalence and prognostic value of cutaneous manifestations in patients with myelodysplastic syndrome. Journal of the European Academy of Dermatology and Venereology. 2010; **24**(10):1171-1175

[65] Dalamaga M, Karmaniolas K, Matekovits A, Migdalis I, Papadavid E. Cutaneous manifestations in relation to immunologic parameters in a cohort of primary myelodysplastic syndrome patients. Journal of the European Academy of Dermatology and Venereology. 2008;**22**(5):543-548

[66] Okamoto T, Okada M, Mori A, Saheki K, Takatsuka H, Wada H, et al. Correlation between immunological abnormalities and prognosis in myelodysplastic syndrome patients. International Journal of Hematology. 1997;**66**(3):345-351

[67] Giannouli S, Voulgarelis M, Zintzaras E, Tzioufas AG, Moutsopoulos HM. Autoimmune phenomena in myelodysplastic syndromes: A 4-yr prospective study. Rheumatology (Oxford, England). 2004;**43**(5):626-632

[68] Raj K, Ho A, Creamer JD, du Vivier AW, Salisbury JR, Mufti GJ. Complete response of deep neutrophilic dermatosis associated with myelodysplastic syndrome to 5-azacytidine. The British Journal of Dermatology. 2007;**156**(5):1039-1041

[69] Pilorge S, Doleris LM, Dreyfus F, Park S. The autoimmune manifestations associated with myelodysplastic syndrome respond to 5-azacytidine: A report on three cases. British Journal of Haematology. 2011;**153**(5):664-665

[70] Mekinian A, Grignano E, Braun T, Decaux O, Liozon E, Costedoat-Chalumeau N, et al. Systemic inflammatory and autoimmune manifestations associated with

myelodysplastic syndromes and chronic myelomonocytic leukaemia: A French multicentre retrospective study. Rheumatology (Oxford, England). 2016; **55**(2):291-300

[71] Fraison JB, Mekinian A, Grignano E, Kahn JE, Arlet JB, Decaux O, et al. Efficacy of Azacitidine in autoimmune and inflammatory disorders associated with myelodysplastic syndromes and chronic myelomonocytic leukemia. Leukemia Research. 2016;**43**:13-17

[72] Mekinian A, Dervin G, Lapidus N, Kahn JE, Terriou L, Liozon E, et al. GFM, SNFMI, CRI and MINHEMON. Biologics in myelodysplastic syndrome-related systemic inflammatory and autoimmune diseases: French multicenter retrospective study of 29 patients. Autoimmunity Reviews. 2017; **16**(9):903-910

Chapter 4

Immune Dysregulation in MDS: The Role of Cytokines and Immune Cells

Selma D'Silva, Sunil B. Rajadhyaksha and Meenakshi Singh

Abstract

Myelodysplastic syndrome (MDS) is a hematopoietic stem cell disorder affecting individuals over the age of 60 years. It is characterized by ineffective hematopoiesis and extensive apoptosis of hematopoietic cells. MDS patients are at a high risk of transforming in to acute myeloid leukemia. The main cause of apoptosis and escape from immune surveillance in MDS is immune dysregulation caused by a number of factors such as aberrant cytokine production and influence of various immune cells. In the past decade various pro-inflammatory cytokines and a number of immune cells such as Natural Killer cells, regulatory T cells, cytotoxic T cells, mesenchymal stem cells, myeloid derived suppressor cells and dendritic cells have been implicated in immune dysregulation leading to MDS pathogenesis. In this review we focus on the current data available on the role of these immune factors.

Keywords: myelodysplastic syndrome, cytokines, natural killer cells, dendritic cells, mesenchymal derived stem cells

1. Introduction

Myelodysplastic syndrome (MDS) is a group of clonal hematopoietic stem cell disorders with ineffective hematopoiesis, cytopenias and risk of transformation to acute myeloid leukemia (AML). Incidence of MDS is higher in older individuals (>70 years of age) [1, 2]. The severity of MDS could range from indolent disease in which no blood transfusion is required, to borderline AML. An individual can get MDS either de novo, secondary to other myeloid disorders or MDS related to therapy. There are several point mutations associated with MDS [3–5]. Few of the individuals carrying these point mutations have a risk of developing MDS in the future but the factors involved in progression of the disease have not yet been identified [6]. MDS is a multifactorial disorder arising due to factors such as genetic alterations, epigenetic changes, gene transcription dysregulation and immune dysregulation [7]. This chapter is a review of the current data available indicating the role of immune cells in immune dysregulation related to MDS pathogenesis.

IntechOpen

2. Classification of MDS

In 1982, the French-American-British (FAB) classification was established for categorizing various MDS cases. According to this classification, all MDS patients were classified into one of the five groups based on the number of myeloblasts present in the bone marrow: refractory anemia, refractory anemia with ring sideroblasts, chronic myeloid leukemia, refractory anemia in excess of blasts (RAEB), and RAEB in transformation (RAEB-T) [8]. This was then later modified into the World Health Organization (WHO) classification which consists of the following groups: Refractory cytopenia with unilineage dysplasia (RCUD), Refractory anemia with ringed sideroblasts (RARS), Refractory anemia with multilineage dysplasia(RAMD), Refractory anemia with excess blasts-1 (RAEB-1), Refractory anemia with excess blasts-2 (RAEB-2), Unclassified myelodysplastic syndrome (MDS-U), MDS associated with isolated deletion 5q, and Refractory cytopenia of childhood (RCC). Various prognostic scoring systems are used in clinical practice to predict overall survival and risk of transformation to AML in MDS patients. Currently, the International Prognostic Scoring System (IPSS) is used for risk stratification and treatment decision making. This system divides MDS patients into 4 different risk categories: low risk, intermediate-1 risk, intermediate-2 risk and high risk, based on the number of cytopenias, the percentage of blasts and cytogenetics [9].

3. Immune dysregulation in MDS

Immune cells are typically involved in immune surveillance, however, they also play a role in disease progression. Many studies have highlighted the role of different immune cells in immune dysregulation leading to pathogenesis of MDS and progression of disease to AML (**Table 1**). These factors could range from aberrant cytokine levels, increased T helper and cytotoxic cells, lower number of regulatory T cells, and dysfunctional Natural Killer (NK) cells among others.

In MDS there is an imbalance in cell production and apoptosis of aberrant cells. The main feature of MDS is high rate of apoptosis leading to cytopenia. The disturbed immune system leads to cytopenia by not only killing the tumor cells but also normal hematopoietic precursors. The immune dysregulation mechanisms vary between the low-risk and high-risk MDS patients, wherein, low risk patients show a high rate of apoptosis resulting from an immune system that is in an activated proinflammatory state, and in high risk patients there is increase in clonality of the tumor cells which escape immune surveillance resulting in a more immunosuppressive environment [7].

Innate immune cells such as cytokines and NK cells and T cells of the adaptive immunity play a major role in immunosurveillance. Since, immunosurveillance maintains the homeostasis as well as removes the aberrant cells any error in the immune regulatory pathways can lead to cancer [31]. The major cause of escape of immune surveillance in MDS is dysregulation of the immune mechanisms which involves various immune cells (**Figure 1**).

3.1 Role of cytokines in immune dysregulation in MDS

Cytokines and chemokines are soluble low-molecular-weight proteins secreted by immune cells that mediate inflammatory responses and regulate hematopoiesis by modulating bone marrow microenvironment. These are essential for the viability, proliferation and differentiation of hematopoietic stem cells. The lymphoid tissues host the effector lymphocytes in their nascent form. Upon stimulation by chemokines released by the macrophages, the lymphocytes secrete pro-inflammatory cytokines such as IL-2, IFN-gamma, IL-17 and TNF-alpha. Additionally, cytokines such as IL-10 and TGF-Beta are also secreted which down regulate the immune

Sr. No.	Immune factor	Levels	Results	References
1	TNF-α	High	Increased rate of apoptosis	[10]
2	IL2	High	Higher levels in advanced stage MDS as compared to early stage	[11]
3	IL6, GM-CSF	High	Higher levels in advanced stage MDS as compared to early stage	[12]
4	TNF-α	High	Lower overall survival and lower event free survival	[13]
5	TNF-α	Low (<10 pg./ml)	Better overall survival and better progression free survival	[14]
6	CD_4^+ and CD_8^+	Low	Response to immunosuppressive therapy	[15]
7	CD_3^+ and CD_8^+	Low	frequent infections, lower overall survival and transformation into AML	[16]
8	CD_8^+ T cells	High	Inhibition of hematopoiesis	[17, 18]
9	CTLA-4	High	Suppression of T cell activity, escape from immune surveillance, resistance to immunotherapy	[19]
10	CTL's	High	Impairment of immune surveillance and disease progression	[20]
11	MDSC's	High	Inefficient hematopoiesis	[21]
12	MSC's	High	Increased apoptosis, immunosuppression and reduced hematopoiesis	[22]
13	MSC's	High	Poor potential for inhibition of DC differentiation and maturation in low-risk MDS patients	[10]
14	DC's	Abnormalities	Escape of tumor cell from immune recognition, Higher rate of relapse after HSCT	[23]
15	IFN-γ producing NK Cells	Low	Decreased cytolytic function leading to increased tumor load	[24]
16	$CD56^{dim}CD16^+$ NK cells	High	Dysregulation of immune surveillance and ineffective hematopoiesis	[25]
17	Tregs	Low	Defective immune activation and decreased immune surveillance	[26, 27]
18	Tregs	Low	T cell cytotoxicity leading to increased apoptosis in low risk MDS	[28]
19	Tregs	High	Impaired antineoplastic immunity and immune suppression in High risk MDS	[15, 28, 29]
20	Th22 (IL22 producing T cells)	High	Increased apoptosis in high risk MDS patients	[30]

TNF-α: tumor necrosis factor-alpha; IL-2: interleukin-2, IL6: interleukin 6, GM-CSF: granulocyte macrophage colony-stimulating factor, CD4+: cluster of differentiation 4, CD8+: cluster of differentiation 8, CD3+: cluster of differentiation 3, CTLA-4: cytotoxic T-lymphocyte-associated antigen 4, CTL's: cytotoxic T lymphocytes, MDSC's: marrow derived stem cells, MSC's: mesenchymal stem cells, DC's: dendritic cells, IFN-γ: interferon gamma, NK: natural killer, CD56: cluster of differentiation 56, CD16: cluster of differentiation 16, Tregs: T regulatory cells.

Table 1.
The role of various immune cells in MDS pathogenesis.

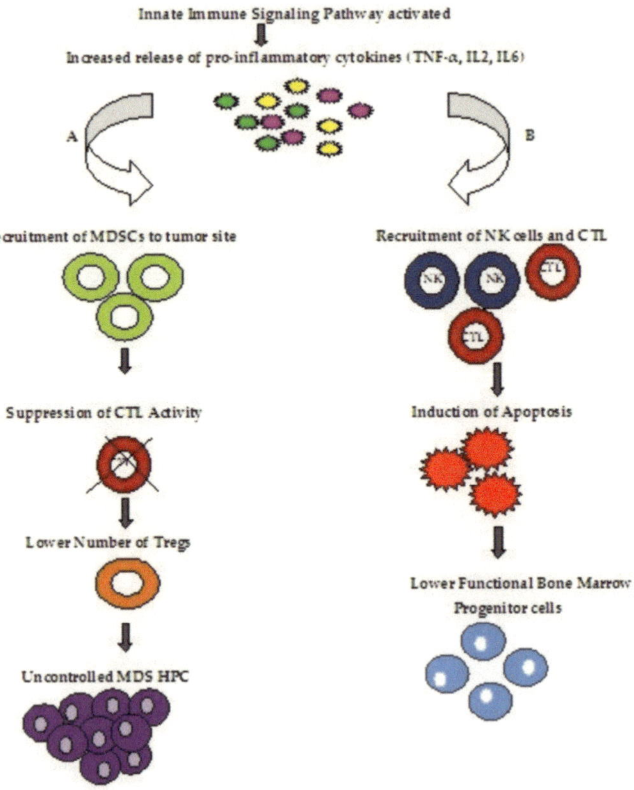

Figure 1.
The role of various immune cells in MDS pathogenesis. **A.** *The abnormal proliferation of MDS hematopoietic cells. The increased release of various pro-inflammatory cytokines directs the recruitment of MDSC's at the tumor site. These kill the erythroid precursor cells and also lead to suppression of CTL activity. Lower number of Tregs enables the tumor cells to escape immune surveillance and leads to accumulation of uncontrolled proliferation of MDS cells.* **B.** *The decrease in normal hematopoiesis. The release of cytokines also leads to increase in the number of natural killer and cytotoxic T cells, which induces apoptosis in hematopoietic stem cells. This in turn results in lower number of functional bone marrow progenitor cells. TNF-α: tumor necrosis factor-alpha, IL2: interleukin-2, IL6: interleukin-6, MDSC: marrow derived stem cells, CTL: cytotoxic T cells, Tregs: regulatory T cells, MDS: mesenchymal stem cells, HPC: hematopoietic cells, NK: natural killer.*

response and contribute in healing the tissue involved. TGF-Beta is also an inducer of regulatory T cells (Tregs). Cytokines such as TNF-alpha have been associated with pathogenesis of high risk MDS, however, their prognostic value is unknown.

One of the causes of cytopenia in MDS is abnormal apoptosis. The increased expression of cytokines such as TNF-alpha, upregulates the expression of cell surface protein Fas receptor. This Fas receptor when bound to its cognate Fas ligand triggers apoptosis of the cell carrying the Fas receptor via the Fas associated death domain (FADD). Hence higher levels of TNF-alpha have been associated with rate of apoptosis in MDS patients [27].

Abnormal levels of cytokines, chemokines and growth factors in MDS patients have been reported by various researchers [32–34]. The levels of pro-inflammatory cytokines such as TNF-alpha, IFN-gamma, TGF-Beta, IL6, IL8, and granulocyte-CSF have been shown to be increased in MDS patients, highlighting the role of these immune cells in immune dysregulation related to MDS [33, 35–39]. Kornblau et al. [40] reported that MDS patients have lower levels of pleiotropic cytokines IL10 and IL4 as compared to healthy controls. Zoumbos et al. [11] have reported higher serum IL2 levels in patients with advanced MDS as compared to early stage patients. Similarly, higher serum IL6 and GM-CSF levels have been reported in patients with advanced MDS [12]. Verhoef et al. [34] have also reported higher levels of IL-3, IL-6 and G-CSF in patients with MDS as compared to controls.

Aberrant cytokine levels have also been associated with MDS clinical outcomes. Tsimberidou et al. [13] have associated higher levels of leukocytes and lower levels of hemoglobin with lower overall survival and event free survival in high-risk MDS patients having higher TNF-alpha levels. Meyers et al. [41] have associated higher levels of TNF-alpha, IL-6, IL-1R with fatigue in MDS patients. Low TNF-alpha (<10 pg./ml) have been associated with better overall survival and better progression free survival [14]. Pardanani et al. [42] suggested the levels of IL6, IL7 and CXCL10 to be an independent prognostic factor for overall survival, wherein, patients with normal levels of these cytokines show better overall survival as compared to those with elevated levels of at least 1.

Lopes et al. [43] reported difference in cytokine profiles between low and high risk MDS cases. Also an inverse relation between IL10 and CD_8^+ T cells has been reported and IL10 expression is much higher in patients suffering from MDS. When comparing the MDS according to the risk, patients in the low risk group show elevated levels of type I cytokines such as IL-1Beta, IL7, IL8 and IL12, whereas high-risk MDS patients show elevated levels of inhibitory factors such as IL10 and sIL2 [13, 14]. Since low-risk MDS is associated with higher apoptotic rates, the levels of cytokines such as TNF-alpha, IFN-gamma and IL-6 are higher in these patients as compared to high-risk MDS patients [35]. High risk MDS is associated with escape of tumor clones from immune recognition and hence serum of these patients have higher amounts of immunosuppressive cytokines like IL10 [44]. IFN-gamma and IL-6 are involved in apoptosis induction in BM. Hence, when they are present in higher levels, it will result in a low risk MDS [27, 32].

4. Role of immune cells

4.1 Helper and cytotoxic T cells

Cytotoxic T cells (CTLs) are cells that are capable of killing cancer cells and abnormal cells. Most of these cells have a T cell receptor (TCR) that recognizes specific antigens, hence, stimulating an immune response. Functionally stable TCRs are associated with both CD_4^+ and CD_8^+ glycoproteins. CD_4^+ glycoproteins are found on cells such as dendritic cells (DC), T helper cells, etc. and are involved in communicating with antigen presenting cells (APCs). The CD_8^+ glycoprotein is present in various cytotoxic cells such as CTL, NK cells etc. Function of CD_8^+ glycoprotein is to recognize and destroy foreign/infectious particles. Only when the TCR is associated with CD_8^+ glycoprotein can it bind to the specific antigens and enable presentation and destruction of these foreign antigens [45, 46].

Growth of both malignant and non-malignant cells in MDS is inhibited by CD_8^+ T cells that target MHC class I molecules on the hematopoietic precursors. This response forms part of the immune surveillance. Majority of MDS patients have peripheral blood lymphopenia, which results in reduction of CD_4^+ and CD_8^+ cell, leading to an inverted CD_4/CD_8 ratio in these patients. In younger patients there is a decrease in both naïve CD_4^+ and CD_8^+ T cells which is also correlated with response to immunosuppressive treatments [15].

The distribution of CD_8^+ T cells differs between low and high risk MDS patients. Low risk MDS patients usually show downregulated Tregs and upregulated CD_8^+ T cells, whereas, high risk MDS patients have upregulated Tregs and downregulated CD_8^+ T cells and NK cells. Symeonidis et al. [16] have reported association of CD_3^+ and CD_8^+ lymphopenia in MDS patients with frequent infections, lower overall survival and transformation into AML. Smith et al. [17] demonstrated inhibition of hematopoiesis by CD_8^+ T cells. This inhibition due to type-I polarization of CD_4^+ and CD_8^+ T cells was also confirmed by Wu et al. in 2008 [18].

Recently, a few epitopes on CD_8^+ T cells such as Wilms tumor 1 protein (WT1), MHC Class I etc., have been implicated in activation of the CD_8^+ T cells. Sloand et al. [47] reported that in MDS patients with trisomy 8, WT1 is highly overexpressed on CD_{34}^+ T cells making these patients more responsive to immunosuppressive therapies. However, these immunosuppressive therapies hinder tumor surveillance by T cells resulting in disease progression.

Further, molecules such as programmed death 1 (PD1), its ligand PD1L, and T cell associated antigen CTLA-4 suppress T cell activity leading to escape of tumor cells from immune surveillance and resistance to immunotherapy [19]. Sand et al. [20] have reported a higher number of CTL's in high-risk MDS patients, however, these CTL's have a lower TCR mediated cytotoxicity, which results in impairment of immune surveillance and leads to disease progression.

A Japanese study revealed lower marrow T cells in MDS-RAEB patients and low $CD_4^+CD45RA^+$ naïve cells in MDS patients indicating impaired immune surveillance and expansion of the tumor clone [48]. Hamdi et al. [49] reported higher Th1/Th2 ratios in patients with lower risk prognostic score. Li et al. [50] have reported higher T cell count in low-risk MDS patients as compared to high-risk patients and controls.

These studies highlight the role of abnormal helper and cytotoxic T cells in autoimmunity towards hematopoietic progenitors.

4.2 Myeloid derived suppressor cells (MDSC's)

Myeloid derived suppressor cells (MDSC's) are cells belonging to the innate immunity involved in suppression of the immune system. These cells express CD33 immune receptor [51]. They are generally in few numbers in healthy individuals but increase in response to stress stimuli. They have been reported in higher frequencies in various cancers.

MDSC's are one of the cells that inhibit anti-tumor immunity. These can be differentiated based on the surface markers as monocytic (MO-MDSC) and granulocytic (PMN-MSDC). The surface markers on monocytic MDSC's are $CD11b^+CD14^+CD15^-CD33^+$ and $HLA\text{-}DR^{low}$, whereas, those on granulocytic MDSC's are $CD11b^+CD14^-CD15^+CD33^+$ and $HLA\text{-}DR^{low/-}$. MDSC's are generally induced by the pro-inflammatory nature of the tumor cells. Their function is to inhibit both adaptive as well as the innate immune system by either cell–cell contact or by releasing cytokines, which results in the inhibition of T cell proliferation and activation, induction of Tregs and NK cell impairment. MDSC's are also involved in inhibiting T cells to settle in the lymph nodes and inflammation sites. MDSC's derived from monocytes and granulocytes support tumor by releasing growth factors.

There is sparing data available regarding the role of MDSC in MDS. The increase in MDSC's in MDS patient results in suppression of normal hematopoiesis and leads to progression of the disease. Chen et al. [21], reported an association of inefficient hematopoiesis with increased MDSC's in the bone marrow of patients with MDS. Graft versus host disease (GvHD) is the number one cause of morbidity and mortality following allogeneic hematopoietic stem cell transplantation. Low levels of MO-MDSC's have been reported in association with onset of aGvHD [52]. The levels of both MO-MDSCs and PMN-MDSCs are increased in the peripheral blood soon after transplant and are reported to lower the risk of acute GvHD (aGvHD) as well as response to steroid therapy [53].

Lechner et al. [54], reported the role of various cytokines in the development of MDSC's. In MDS there are irregular levels of cytokines which indicates that targeting the cytokine levels can lead to loss of immunosuppression by the MDSC's. Jiang et al. [55], reported increased levels of circulating MDSC's in MDS patients. The immature myeloid cells induce secretion of cytokines such as IL-10 and TGF-Beta which increase the levels of MDSC's.

4.3 Mesenchymal stem cells

MSC's are self-renewing cells with the ability to differentiate into a number of cells such as adipocytes, and chondrocytes. The main role of MSC's is maintaining normal hematopoiesis, however, they are also implicated in MDS pathogenesis. The role of MSC's in MDS is different in low risk and high-risk patients. In high risk patients MSC's induce apoptosis and suppress the immune system by secreting various cytokines like TGF-B, whereas, in low risk patients they reduce the efficiency for inhibiting DC differentiation. Since MSC's have an immunomodulatory role, they have been investigated for their role in MDS disease progression. However, most of the studies have reported contradictory results and a consensus on the involvement of MSC's in MDS is not yet sought.

Han et al. [56] have demonstrated MSC's with normal morphology and phenotype, but with deficient immunomodulatory function that could not inhibit in vitro T cell activation and proliferation. Klaus et al. [57], did not find any difference in the differentiation potential and immunosuppressive potential of MSC's in MDS patients and controls. In high-risk MDS patients, Zhao et al. [22] reported MSC's with an increase in apoptosis, immunosuppressive rate and reduced hematopoiesis, whereas, Wang et al. [10] reported MSC's with poor potential for inhibition of DC differentiation and maturation in low-risk MDS patients.

4.4 Dendritic cells

The site of origin of DC's is the bone marrow. There are four different types of dendritic cells present in the peripheral blood: plasmacytoid DCs (pDCs), two types of myeloid DCs and slan DC's. The main function of DC's is pathogen and tumor recognition and antigen presentation [58, 59]. Hence, any defect in DC's could mean that the tumor cells will escape immune recognition [28, 29]. DC's upregulate and activate co-receptors on T cells. In MDS patients the ability of DC's to activate T cells is much lower as compared to healthy controls [60]. Ma et al. [61], reported similarities in cytogenetic abnormalities in DC's of MDS patients and in their malignant clones indicating that these abnormalities belonged to the malignant clone.

DC's are equipped with Toll-like receptors and C-type lectin receptors which help in recognition of pathogens. DC's are usually in a nascent state and upon contact with potential pathogens they mature. During maturation there are morphological changes due to which the function of DC's changes from pathogen capturing to cytokine secretion and antigen presentation. The processed antigens on MHC's are presented by DC's to naïve T cells which then elicit an immune response.

Various researchers have reported aberrant immune response by DC's in different cancer types [62–66]. This defect could be in the frequency of DC's, maturation, cytokine secretion profile, and ability to induce T cell proliferation [7]. Abnormalities and defects in number of dendritic cells lead to escape of tumor cell from immune recognition, hence, resulting in higher rate of relapse after allogeneic HSCT [23]. The number and frequency of DC's in the peripheral blood of MDS cases is much reduced as compared to healthy individuals [60, 61, 67]. Further their capability to stimulate T cells is also reduced due to lower surface expression of molecules such as CD54, CD80 and CD86 [60]. Ma et al. [68] have reported lower IL12 secretion and higher IL10 secretion in DC's from MDS patients. Saft et al. [23] reported lower myeloid and plasmacytoid precursor DC's in high-risk MDS as compared to low-risk MDS patients.

4.5 Natural killer cells

Natural Killer cells (NK) play an important role in innate immunity. NK cells secrete cytokines and play an important role in host defense [69]. Their main role is to kill non-self cells, i.e., cells that lack self-major histocompatibility complex (MHC). NK cell cytotoxicity can either be activated or inhibited based on the sum of the activating and inhibitory receptors present on their surface. The inhibitory receptors could either be Killer immunoglobulin like receptors (KIR) or CD94/NKG2A dimer which protect self-cells from NK cell lysis by binding to their cognate MHC Class I ligands [70], whereas, the activating receptors are the natural cytotoxic receptors (NCRs), namely, NKp46, NKp44, NKp30 and NKG2D [69, 71].

The role of NK cells in immune dysregulation in MDS results from reduction in total number or functional NK cells leading to defects in immune surveillance and hence disease progression. Since NK cells eliminate the aberrant cells from the system, deficiency of NK cell functionality has been associated with poor prognosis in MDS, hence, in older patients, where in the NK cell activity is already low due to aging, the NK cell activity decreases further.

Various reports have measured NK cells in MDS patients [72–74]. Epling-Burnette et al., reported 2 types of NK cells based in their cytotoxicity: low function NK cells which have been associated with high-risk MDS, and normal function NK cells. Furthermore, they also reported defects in number of activating NK receptors such as NKG2D leading to progression of disease. They observed reduced NK cell cytolytic activity in MDS patients as compared to healthy donors. The activating receptors NKp30 and NKG2D was downregulated in these patients [74].

Fujii et al. [24], reported deficiency of IFN-gamma producing NK T cells in blood and marrow of MDS patients. This led to decreased cytolytic function leading to tumor load. Zhang et al. [25], report lower expression of $CD3^{-}CD56^{+}CD16^{+}$ NK cells in MDS patients as compared to healthy individuals. $CD16^{+}$ NK cells play an important role in tumor surveillance, and hence decreased count of these cells correlate with the tumor cell load in MDS patients [75, 76].

$CD56^{+}$ is a marker for NK cells that produce high levels of cytokines. Circulating NK cells usually exhibit $CD56^{dim}$ which produce lower amounts of cytokines as compared to $CD56^{bright}$ NK cells. Hence, $CD56^{bright}$ are known to have a more immunomodulatory role as compared to $CD56^{dim}$ which are mostly cytotoxic in nature [77]. In patients with MDS, there is a higher prevalence of $CD56^{dim}CD16^{+}$ cells as compared to healthy controls which results in dysregulation of immune surveillance and ineffective hematopoiesis [25]. Hejazi et al. [72] conducted a study on 75 MDS patients, wherein it was observed that majority of the patients in the high risk group had a NK Cell deficiency, moreover, in another group, it was observed that although NK cells were present, they were non-functional. $CD56^{dim}$ NK cells were predominantly present which result in reduction of cytotoxicity.

4.6 Regulatory T cells

Tregs are T helper cells that are involved in immune tolerance and modulation of immune reactions. Regulatory T cells (Tregs) cells are $CD4^{+}CD25^{high}FOXP3^{+}$ or $CD4^{+}CD25^{high}CD127^{low}$. Tregs carry out immune tolerance as well as modulation of immune response and are the important for immune surveillance [27] by secreting IL10 and TGF-Beta which are immunosuppressive cytokines [78]. Any impairment in Tregs results in defective immune activation and decreased immune surveillance against the tumor cells [26]. Lower numbers of functional Tregs result in autoimmunity.

The exact role of Tregs in MDS progression is not very clear. However, variation in number of Tregs has been reported to be associated with disease progression, risk of transformation to AML and overall survival in MDS patients [29, 31, 49, 79]. The very first study for the involvement of Tregs in MDS was demonstrated by Kordasti et al. [29], wherein, an association between increased CD_4^+ Tregs and disease progression was shown. Low number of Tregs in bone marrow have been linked to increased CD_8^+ T cells and the recruitment of Th17 proinflammatory cells [44, 80]. The number of Tregs differs based on the disease stage. In low-risk MDS, lower numbers of Tregs or impaired Tregs have been reported in association with T cell cytotoxicity leading to increased apoptosis, whereas, higher number of Tregs are seen in high-risk MDS patients and are associated with impaired antineoplastic immunity and immune suppression [15, 28, 29].

Costantini et al. [81] conducted a study to investigate the effect of 5-azacytidine on Tregs functionality in intermediate/high risk MDS patients. Following treatment, lower numbers and Tregs with lower suppressive function were observed in these patients. Alfinito et al. [80] reported an inverse relationship between levels of Tregs and the degree of dyserythropoiesis. Hamdi et al. [49], reported an inverse ratio between Treg and CD_8^+ frequencies in MDS patients. Low risk MDS patients have higher number of Th17 cells which is inversely correlated with Tregs numbers. Hence in these patients the Th17/Tregs ratio is found to be increased [44]. Shao et al. [30] have shown increased number of Th22 (IL22 producing T cells) in high-risk MDS patients. This increased number of Th22 is correlated with release of pro-inflammatory cytokines leading to increased apoptosis.

5. Immunosuppressive therapy

The most curative treatment for MDS is allogeneic hematopoietic stem cell therapy; however, since MDS develops mostly later in life, most patients are rendered ineligible for transplantation and supportive care is their only option for treatment. As previously discussed, many researchers have shown the involvement of immune cells in the pathogenesis of MDS and hence, immunosuppression involving targeting these cells has evolved as one of the treatment modalities.

Molldrem et al. and Jonasova et al. [82, 83] were the first to report the use of immunosuppressive therapy (IST) in MDS with Antithymoglobulin (ATG) in 1997 and Cyclosporin (CsA) in 1998 respectively. Jonasova et al. [83] reported positive response in MDS-RA patients treated with CsA. On the contrary, another study showed no advantage to CsA and also reported CsA related renal toxicity [84]. CsA acts by blocking IL-2 production which leads to inhibition of expansion of CTLs and suppression of cytokines like TNF-α which are involved in apoptosis [85]. ATG has a role in depleting T cells and restoring normal hematopoiesis [86]. It acts by interfering with the normal function of DC's and hence inhibiting the interaction between the T cell and the antigen presenting cell. Moreover, ATG restores normal hematopoiesis by diminishing cytokine release by activated T cells [87].

Since reduced number of Tregs are associated with disease progression in low-risk MDS, introduction of ex-vivo expanded Tregs is a potential targeted therapy in such patients. Not only the number but also the function of Tregs is important, hence, it is absolutely necessary to be sure that the ex-vivo expanded Tregs population do not have non-regulatory effector cells. Functional Tregs can be also be induced by vaccination using tolerizing DC's [88].

6. Conclusions

It is now well known that genetic, epigenetic and aberrant immune factors play a major role in the pathogenesis of MDS, making it one of the most challenging disorders to design therapies for. Leaving aside the MDS patients in whom the major factor is genetic mutations, there is a group of patients in whom immune cells play a major role in the disease progression. In these patients, immunosuppressive therapies (IST) form part of the major treatment strategy. It is known that there is improved marrow function and increased survival in patients undergoing IST. However, identifying patients that will respond favorably is a challenge. Some targeted therapies involve introducing tolerogenic DC's and expansion of Tregs. The therapeutic approach becomes more difficult because of the difference in the immune environment that exists between low-risk and high-risk MDS cases. For this the exact immune mechanisms involved and the specific immune cells responsible for the pathogenesis in the particular group of patients need to be identified in order to establish targeted therapies in the future.

Conflict of interest

The authors declare that there is no conflict of interest.

Author details

Selma D'Silva, Sunil B. Rajadhyaksha and Meenakshi Singh*
HLA and Immunogenetics Laboratory, Department of Transfusion Medicine, Tata Memorial Hospital, Mumbai, India

*Address all correspondence to: meenakshisingha@gmail.com

References

[1] Greenberg P, Cox C, LeBeau MM, Fenaux P, Morel P, Sanz G, et al. International scoring system for evaluating prognosis in myelodysplastic syndromes. Blood. 1997;**89**:2079-2088

[2] Estey E. Acute myeloid leukemia and myelodysplastic syndromes in older patients. Journal of Clinical Oncology. 2007;**25**:1908-1915. DOI: 10.1200/JCO.2006.10.2731

[3] Kim E, Ilagan JO, Liang Y, Daubner GM, Lee SC, Ramakrishnan A, et al. SRSF2 mutations contribute to myelodysplasia by mutant-specific effects on exon recognition. Cancer Cell. 2015;**27**:617-630. DOI: 10.1016/j.ccell.2015.04.006

[4] Aslan D, Garde C, Nygaard MK, Helbo AS, Dimopoulos K, Hansen JW, et al. Tumor suppressor microRNAs are downregulated in myelodysplastic syndrome with spliceosome mutations. Oncotarget. 2016;**7**:9951-9963. DOI: 10.18632/oncotarget.7127

[5] Treppendahl MB, Kristensen LS, Groønb K. Predicting response to epigenetic therapy. Journal of Clinical Investigations. 2014;**124**:47-55. DOI: 10.1172/JCI69737

[6] Kwok B, Hall JM, Witte JS, Xu Y, Reddy P, Lin K, et al. MDS-associated somatic mutations and clonal hematopoiesis are common in idiopathic cytopenias of undetermined significance. Blood. 2015;**126**:2355-2362. DOI: 10.1182/blood-2015-08-667063

[7] Kerkhoff N, Bontkes HJ, Westers TM, de Gruijl TD, Kordasti S, van de Loosdrecht AA. Dendritic cells in myeloblastic syndromes: From pathogenesis to immunotherapy. Immunotherapy. 2013;**5**(6):621-637. DOI: 10.2217/imt.13.51

[8] Bennett JM, Catovsky D, Daniel MT, Flandrin G, Gralnick HR, Sultan C. Proposals for the classification of the myelodysplastic syndromes. British Journal of Haematology. 1982;**51**:189-199

[9] Sugimori C, List AF, Epling-Burnette PK. Immune dysregulation in myelodysplastic syndrome. Hematology Reports. 2010;**2**:e1. DOI: 10.4081/hr.2010.e1

[10] Wang Z, Tang X, Xu W, Cao Z, Sun L, Li W, et al. The different immunoregulatory functions on dendritic cells between mesenchymal stem cells derived from bone marrow of patients with low risk or high risk myelodysplastic syndromes. PLoS One. 2013;**8**:e57470. DOI: 10.1371/journal.pone.0057470

[11] Zoumbos N, Symeonidis A, Kourakli A, Katevas P, Matsouka P, Perraki M, et al. Increased levels of soluble interleukin-2 receptors and tumor necrosis factor in serum of patients with myelodysplastic syndromes. Blood. 1991;**77**:413-414

[12] Wetzler M, Kurzrock R, Estrov Z, Estey E, Talpaz M. Cytokine expression in adherent layers from patients with myelodysplastic syndrome and acute myelogenous leukemia. Leukemia Research. 1995;**19**:23-34

[13] Tsimberidou AM, Estey E, Wen S, Pierce S, Kantarjian H, Albitar M, et al. The prognostic significance of cytokine levels in newly diagnosed acute myeloid leukemia and high-risk myelodysplastic syndromes. Cancer. 2008;**113**:1605-1613. DOI: 10.1002/cncr.23785

[14] Musto P, Matera R, Minervini MM, Checchia-de AC, Bodenizza C, Falcone A, et al. Low serum levels of tumor necrosis factor and interleukin-1β in myelodysplastic syndromes responsive to recombinant erythropoietin. Haematologica. 1994;**79**:265-268

[15] Zou JX, Rollison DE, Boulware D, Chen DT, Sloand EM, Pfannes LV, et al. Altered naive and memory CD4+ T-cell homeostasis and immunosenescence characterize younger patients with myelodysplastic syndrome. Leukemia. 2009;**23**:1288-1296. DOI: 10.1038/leu.2009

[16] Symeonidis A, Zoumbos N. Defective autologous and allogeneic mixed lymphocyte reaction in patients with primary myelodysplastic syndromes. Leukemia Research. 1991;**15**(suppl. 1):29. DOI: 10.1016/0145-2126(91)90436-W

[17] Smith MA, Smith JG. The occurrence subtype and significance of hematopoietic inhibitory T cells (HIT cells) in myelodysplasia: An invitro study. Leukemia Research. 1991;**15**:597-601

[18] Wu L, Li X, Chang C, Ying S, He Q, Pu Q. Deviation of type I and type II T cells and its negative effect on hematopoeisis in myelodysplastic syndrome. International Journal of Laboratory Hematology. 2008;**30**:390-399. DOI: 10.1111/j.1751-553X.2007.00970.x

[19] Yang H, Bueso-Ramos C, DiNardo C, Estecio MR, Davanlou M, Geng QR, et al. Expression of PD-L1, PD-L2, PD-1 and CTLA4 in myelodysplastic syndromes is enhanced by treatment with hypomethylating agents. Leukemia. 2014;**28**:1280-1288. DOI: 10.1038/leu.2013.355

[20] Sand K, Theorell J, Bruserud O, Bryceson YT, Kittang AO. Reduced potency of cytotoxic T lymphocytes from patients with high-risk myelodysplastic syndromes. Cancer Immunology, Immunotherapy. 2016;**65**(9):1135-1147. DOI: 10.1007/s00262-016-1865-y

[21] Chen X, Eksioglu EA, Zhou J, Zhang L, Djeu J, Fortenbery N, et al. Induction of myelodysplasia by myeloid- derived suppressor cells. Journal of Clinical Investigations. 2013;**123**:4595-4611. DOI: 10.1172/JCI67580

[22] Zhao Z, Wang Z, Li Q, Li W, You Y, Zhou P. The different immunoregulatory functions of mesenchymal stem cells in patients with low-risk or high-risk myelodysplastic syndromes. PLoS One. 2012;**7**:e45675. DOI: 10.1371/journal.pone.0045675

[23] Saft L, Björklund E, Berg E, Hellström-Lindberg E, Porwit A. Bone marrow dendritic cells are reduced in patients with high-risk myelodysplastic syndromes. Leukemia Research. 2013;**37**:266-273. DOI: 10.1016/j.leukres.2012.10.010

[24] Fujii S, Shimizu K, Klimek V, Geller MD, Nimer SD, Dhodapkar MV. Severe and selective deficiency of interferon gamma producing invariant natural killer T cells in patients with myelodysplastic syndromes. British Journal of Hematology. 2003;**122**:617-622

[25] Zhang W, Xie X, Mi H, Sun J, Ding S, Li L, et al. Abnormal populations and functions of natural killer cells in patients with myelodysplastic syndromes. Oncology Letters. 2018;**15**:5497-5504. DOI: 10.3892/ol.2018.8062

[26] Symeonidis A, Kouraklis-symeonidis A. Immune dysregulation in myelodysplastic syndromes: Pathogenetic-pathophysiologic aspects and clinical consequences. In: Fuchs O, editor. Myelodysplastic Syndromes. London: IntechOpen; 2016. DOI: 10.5772/64618. Available from: https://www.intechopen.com/books/myelodysplastic-syndromes/immune-dysregulation-in-myelodysplastic-syndromes-pathogenetic-pathophysiologic-aspects-and-clinical [Accessed: Sep 1, 2018]

[27] Wang C, Wang Y, Gao S, Chen J, Yu J, Zhang H, et al. Immune dysregulation in myelodysplastic syndrome: Clinical features, pathogenesis and therapeutic strategies. Critical Reviews in Oncology/Hematology. 2018;**122**:123-132. DOI: 10.1016/j.critrevonc.2017.12.013

[28] Kotsianidis I, Bouchliou I, Nakou E, Spanoudakis E, Margaritis D, Christophoridou AV, et al. Kinetics, function and bone marrow trafficking of $CD4^+CD25^+FOXP3^+$ regulatory T cells in myelodysplastic syndromes (MDS). Leukemia. 2009;**23**:510-518. DOI: 10.1038/leu.2008.333

[29] Kordasti SY, Ingram W, Hayden J, Darling D, Barber L, Afzali B, et al. $CD4^+CD25^{high}Foxp3^+$ regulatory T cells in myelodysplastic syndrome (MDS). Blood. 2007;**110**(3):847-850. DOI: 10.1182/blood-2007-01-067546

[30] Shao LL, Zhang L, Hou Y, Yu S, Liu XG, Huang XY, et al. Th22 cells as well as Th17 cells expand differentially in patients with early-stage and late-stage myelodysplastic syndrome. PLoS One. 2012;7:e51339. DOI: 10.1371/journal.pone.0051339

[31] Lambert C, Wu Y, Aanei C. Bone marrow immunity and myelodysplasia. Frontiers in Oncology. 2016;**6**:172. DOI: 10.3389/fonc.2016.00172

[32] Gañán-Gómez I, Wei Y, Starczynowski DT, Colla S, Yang H, Cabrero-Calvo M, et al. Deregulation of innate immune and inflammatory signaling in myelodysplastic syndromes. Leukemia. 2015;**29**:1458-1469. DOI: 10.1038/leu.2015.69

[33] Kitagawa M, Saito I, Kuwata T, Yoshida S, Yamaguchi S, Takahashi M, et al. Overexpression of tumor necrosis factor (TNF)-α and interferon (IFN)-gamma by bone marrow cells from patients with myelodysplastic syndromes. Leukemia. 1997;**11**:2049-2054

[34] Verhoef GE, De Schouwer P, Ceuppens JL, Van Damme J, Goossens W, Boogaerts MA. Measurement of serum cytokine levels in patients with myelodysplastic syndromes. Leukemia. 1992;**6**:1268-1272

[35] Shetty V, Mundle S, Alvi S, Showel M, Broady-Robinson L, Dar S, et al. Measurement of apoptosis, proliferation and three cytokines in 46 patients with myelodysplastic syndromes. Leukemia Research. 1996;**20**:891-900

[36] Allampallam K, Shetty V, Hussaini S, Mazzoran L, Zorat F, Huang R, et al. Measurement of mRNA expression for a variety of cytokines and its receptors in bone marrows of patients with myelodysplastic syndromes. Anticancer Research. 1999;**19**:5323-5328

[37] Gersuk GM, Beckham C, Loken MR, Kiener P, Anderson JE, Farrand A, et al. A role for tumour necrosis factor-alpha, Fas and Fas-ligand in marrow failure associated with myelodysplastic syndrome. British Journal of Haematology. 1998;**103**:176-188

[38] Sawanobori M, Yamaguchi S, Hasegawa M, Inoue M, Suzuki K, Kamiyama R, et al. Expression of TNF receptors and related signaling molecules in the bone marrow from patients with myelodysplastic syndromes. Leukemia Research. 2003;**27**:583-591

[39] Hsu HC, Lee YM, Tsai WH, Jiang ML, Ho CH, Ho CK, et al. Circulating levels of thrombopoietic and inflammatory cytokines in patients with acute myeloblastic leukemia and myelodysplastic syndrome. Oncology. 2002;**63**:64-69. DOI: 10.1159/000065722

[40] Kornblau SM, McCue D, Singh N, Chen W, Estrov Z, Coombes KR. Recurrent expression signatures of cytokines and chemokines are present and are independently prognostic in acute myelogenous

leukemia and myelodysplasia. Blood. 2010;**116**:4251-4261. DOI: 10.1182/blood-2010-01-262071

[41] Meyers CA, Albitar M, Estey E. Cognitive impairment, fatigue, and cytokine levels in patients with acute myelogenous leukemia or myelodysplastic syndrome. Cancer. 2005;**104**:788-793. DOI: 10.1002/cncr.21234

[42] Pardanani A, Finke C, Lasho TL, Al-Kali A, Begna KH, Hanson CA, et al. IPSS independent prognostic value of plasma CXCL10, IL-7 and IL-6 levels in myelodysplastic syndromes. Leukemia. 2012;**26**:693-699. DOI: 10.1038/leu.2011.251

[43] Lopes MR, Traina F, Campos Pde M, Pereira JK, Machado-Neto JA, Machado Hda C, et al. IL10 inversely correlates with the percentage of CD8+ cells in MDS patients. Leukemia Research. 2013;**37**:541-546. DOI: 10.1016/j.leukres.2013.01.019

[44] Kordasti SY, Afzali B, Lim Z, Ingram W, Hayden J, Barber L, et al. IL-17-producing CD4(+) T cells, pro-inflammatory cytokines and apoptosis are increased in low risk myelodysplastic syndrome. British Journal of Haematology. 2009;**145**:64-72. DOI: 10.1111/j.1365-2141.2009.07593.x

[45] Bernard A, Boumsell L, Hill C. Joint report of the first international workshop on human leucocyte differentiation antigens by the investigators of the participating laboratories. In: Bernard A, Boumsell L, Dausset J, Milstein C, Schlossman SF, editors. Leucocyte Typing: Human Leucocyte Differentiation Antigens Detected by Monoclonal Antibodies: Specification, Classification, Nomenclature. Berlin: Springer; 1984. pp. 45-48

[46] Leong AS, Cooper K, Leong FJ. Manual of Diagnostic Cytology. 2nd ed. Cambridge: Greenwich Medical Media, Ltd; 2003. 73 p

[47] Sloand EM, Melenhorst JJ, Tucker ZC, Pfannes L, Brenchley JM, Yong A, et al. T cell immune responses to Wilms tumor 1 protein in myelodysplasia responsive to immunosuppressive therapy. Blood 2011;**117**:2691-2699. DOI: 10.1182/blood-2010-04-277921

[48] Iwase O, Aizawa S, Kuriyama Y, Yaguchi M, Nakano M, Toyama K. Analysis of bone marrow and peripheral blood immunoregulatory lymphocytes in patients with myelodysplastic syndrome. Annals of Hematology. 1995;**71**:293-299

[49] Hamdi W, Ogawara H, Handa H, Tsukamoto N, Murakami H. Clinical significance of Th1/Th2 ratio in patients with myelodysplastic syndrome. International Journal of Laboratory Hematology. 2009;**31**:630-638. DOI: 10.1111/j.1751-553X.2008.01090.x

[50] Li X, Xu F, He Q, Wu L, Zhang Z, Chang C. Comparison of immunological abnormalities of lymphocytes in bone marrow in myelodysplastic syndrome (MDS) and aplastic anemia (AA). Internal Medicine. 2010;**49**:1349-1355

[51] Gabrilovich DI, Nagaraj S. Myeloid-derived suppressor cells as regulators of the immune system. Nature Reviews Immunology. 2009;**9**:162-174. DOI: 10.1038/nri2506

[52] Lv M, Zhao XS, Hu Y, Chang YJ, Zhao XY, Kong Y, et al. Monocytic and promyelocytic myeloid derived suppressor cells may contribute to G-CSF-induced immune tolerance in haplo-identical allogeneic hematopoietic stem cell transplanatation. American Journal of Hematology. 2015;**90**(1):E9-E16. DOI: 10.1002/ajh.23865.

[53] Beckers M, Dierickx D, Devos T, Fevery S, Sprangers B. The role of myeloid-derived suppressor cells in haematology: Hype or reality? Belgian Journal of Hematology. 2016;**7**(6):213-216

[54] Lechner MG, Liebertz DJ, Epstein AL. Characterization of cytokine induced myeloid derived suppressor cells from normal human peripheral blood mononuclear cells. Journal of Immunology. 2010;**185**:2273-2284. DOI: 10.4049/jimmunol.1000901

[55] Jiang HJ, Fu R, Wang HQ, Li LJ, Qu W, Liang Y, et al. Increased circulating of myeloid derives suppressor cells in myelodysplastic syndrome. Chinese Medical Journal. 2013;**126**:2582-2584

[56] Han Q, Sun Z, Liu L, Chen B, Cao Y, Li K, et al. Impairement in immune-modulatory function of Flk1(+)CD31(−)CD34(−) MSCs from MDS-RA patients. Leukemia Research. 2007;**31**:1469-1478. DOI: 10.1016/j.leukres.2006.12.016

[57] Klaus M, Stavroulaki E, Kastrinaki MC, Fragioudaki P, Giannikou K, Psyllaki M, et al. Reserves, functional, immunoregulatory, and cytogenetic properties of bone marrow mesenchymal stem cells in patients with myelodysplastic syndromes. Stem Cells Development. 2010;**19**:1043-1054. DOI: 10.1089/scd.2009.0286

[58] Banchereau J, Steinman RM. Dendritic cells and the control of immunity. Nature. 1998;**392**(6673): 245-252. DOI: 10.1038/32588

[59] Banchereau J, Briere F, Caux C, Davoust J, Lebecque S, Liu YJ, et al. Immunobiology of dendritic cells. Annual Review of Immunology. 2000;**1**:767-811. DOI: 10.1146/annurev.immunol.18.1.767

[60] Matteo Rigolin G, Howard J, Buggins A, Sneddon C, Castoldi G, Hirst WJ, et al. Phenotypic and functional characteristics of monocyte-derived dendritic cells from patients with myelodysplastic syndromes. British Journal of Haematology. 1999;**107**:844-850

[61] Ma L, Delforge M, van Duppen V, Verhoef G, Emanuel B, Boogaerts M, et al. Circulating myeloid and lymphoid precursor dendritic cells are clonally involved in myelodysplastic syndromes. Leukemia. 2004;**18**:1451-1456. DOI: 10.1038/sj.leu.2403430

[62] Gabrilovich D. Mechanisms and functional significance of tumour-induced dendritic-cell defects. Nature Reviews Immunology. 2004;**4**(12):941-952. DOI: 10.1038/nri1498

[63] Hoffmann TK, Müller-Berghaus J, Ferris RL, Johnson JT, Storkus WJ, Whiteside TL. Alterations in the frequency of dendritic cell subsets in the peripheral circulation of patients with squamous cell carcinomas of the head and neck. Clinical Cancer Research. 2002;**8**:1787-1793

[64] Della Bella S, Gennaro M, Vaccari M, Ferraris C, Nicola S, Riva A, et al. Altered maturation of peripheral blood dendritic cells in patients with breast cancer. British Journal of Cancer. 2003;**89**(8):1463-1472. DOI: 10.1038/sj.bjc.6601243

[65] Dong R, Cwynarski K, Entwistle A, Marelli-Berg F, Dazzi F, Simpson E, et al. Dendritic cells from CML patients have altered actin organization, reduced antigen processing, and impaired migration. Blood. 2003;**101**(9):3560-3567. DOI: 10.1182/blood-2002-06-1841

[66] Mohty M. Circulating blood dendritic cells from myeloid leukemia patients display quantitative and cytogenetic abnormalities as well as functional impairment. Blood. 2001;**98**(13):3750-3756

[67] Micheva I, Thanopoulou E, Michalopoulou S, Karakantza M, Kouraklis-Symeonidis A, Mouzaki A, et al. Defective tumor necrosis factor alpha-induced maturation of monocyte-derived dendritic cells in patients with myelodysplastic syndromes. Clinical

Immunology. 2004;**113**(3):310-317. DOI: 10.1016/j.clim.2004.08.007

[68] Ma L, Ceuppens J, Kasran A, Delforge M, Boogaerts M, Vandenberghe P. Immature and mature monocyte-derived dendritic cells in myelodysplastic syndromes of subtypes refractory anemia or refractory anemia with ringed sideroblasts display an altered cytokine profile. Leukemia Research. 2007;**31**(10):1373-1382. DOI: 10.1016/j.leukres.2006.11.007

[69] Wu J, Lanier LL. Natural killer cells and cancer. Advances in Cancer Research. 2003;**90**:127-156

[70] Uhrberg M, Valiante N, Shum BP, Shilling H, Lienert-Weidenbach K, Corliss B, et al. Human diversity in killer cell inhibitory receptor genes. Immunity. 1997;7:753-763

[71] Miller JS. Biology of natural killer cells in cancer and infection. Cancer Investigations. 2002;**20**:405-419

[72] Hejazi M, Manser AR, Frobel J, Kündgen A, Zhao X, Schönberg K, et al. Impaired cytotoxicity associated with defective natural killer cell differentiation in myelodysplastic syndromes. Haematologica. 2015;**100**:643-652. DOI: 10.3324/haematol.2014.118679

[73] Chamuleau ME, Westers TM, van Dreunen L, Groenland J, Zevenbergen A, Eeltink CM, et al. Immune mediated autologous cytotoxicity against hematopoietic precursor cells in patients with myelodysplastic syndrome. Haematologica. 2009;**94**:496-506. DOI: 10.3324/haematol.13612

[74] Epling-Burnette PK, Bai F, Painter JS, Rollison DE, Salih HR, Krusch M, et al. Reduced natural killer (NK) function associated with high-risk myelodysplastic syndrome (MDS) and reduced expression of activating NK receptors. Blood. 2007;**109**:4816-4824. DOI: 10.1182/blood-2006-07-035519

[75] Konjević G, Mirjacić Martinović K, Jurisić V, Babović N, Spuzić I. Biomarkers of suppressed natural killer (NK) cell function in metastatic melanoma: Decreased NKG2D and increased CD158a receptors on $CD3^{-}CD16^{+}$ NK cells. Biomarkers. 2009;**14**:258-270. DOI: 10.1080/13547500902814658

[76] Ebert LM, Meuter S, Moser B. Homing and function of human skin gammadelta T cells and NK cells: Relevance for tumor surveillance. Journal of Immunology. 2006;**176**:4331-4336

[77] Carlsten M, Baumann BC, Simonsson M. Reduced DNAM-1 expression on bone marrow NK cells associated with impaired killing of CD34(þ) blasts in myelodysplastic syndrome. Leukemia. 2010;**24**:1607-1616. DOI: 10.1038/leu.2010.149

[78] Aggarwal S, van de Loosdrecht, Alhan C, Ossenkoppele GJ, Westers TM, Bontkes HJ. Role of immune responses in the pathogenesis of low risk MDS and high risk MDS: Implications for immunotherapy. British Journal of Hematology. 2011;**153**:568-581. DOI: 10.1111/j.1365-2141.2011.08683.x

[79] Mailloux A, Youn M. Regulatory T-cell trafficking: From thymic development to tumor-induced immune suppression. Critical Reviews in Immunology. 2010;**30**(5):435-447

[80] Alfinito F, Sica M, Luciano L, Della Pepa R, Palladino C, Ferrara I, et al. Immune dysregulation and dyserythropoiesis in the myelodysplastic syndromes. British Journal of Haematology. 2010;**148**:90-98. DOI: 10.1111/j.1365-2141.2009.07921.x

[81] Costantini B, Kordasti SY, Kulasekararaj AG, Jiang J, Seidl T, Abellan PP, et al. The effects of 5-azacytidine on the function and number of regulatory T cells

and T-effectors in myelodysplastic syndrome. Haematologica. 2013;**98**:1196-1205. DOI: 10.3324/haematol.2012.074823

[82] Molldrem JJ, Caples M, Mavroudis D, Plante M, Young NS, Barrett AJ. Antithymocyte globulin for patients with myelodysplastic syndrome. British Journal of Haematology. 1997;**99**:699-705

[83] Jonasova A, Neuwirtova R, Cermak J, Vozobulova V, Mocikova K, Siskova M, et al. Cyclosporin a therapy in hypoplastic MDS patients and certain refractory anaemias without hypoplastic bone marrow. British Journal of Haematology. 1998;**100**:304-309

[84] Atoyebi W, Bywater L, Rawlings L, Brunskill S, Littlewood TJ. Treatment of myelodysplasia with oral cyclosporin. Clinical Laboratory Haematology. 2002;**24**:211-214

[85] Selleri C, Maciejewski JP, Catalano L, Ricci P, Andretta C, Luciano L, et al. Effects of cyclosporine on hematopoietic and immune functions in patients with hypoplastic myelodysplasia: in vitro and in vivo studies. Cancer. 2002;**95**:1911-1922. DOI: 10.1002/cncr.10915

[86] Haidinger M, Geyeregger R, Poglitsch M, Weichhart T, Zeyda M, Vodenik B, et al. Antithymocyte globulin impairs T-cell/antigen-presenting cell interaction: Disruption of immunological synapse and conjugate formation. Transplantation. 2007;**84**:117-121. DOI: 10.1097/01.tp.0000266677.45428.80

[87] Sloand EM, Rezvani K. The role of immune system in myelodysplasia: Implications for therapy. Seminars in Hematology. 2008;**45**:39-48. DOI: 10.1053/j.seminhematol.2007.11.006

[88] Luo X, Tarbell KV, Yang H, Pothoven K, Bailey SL, Ding R, et al. Dendritic cells with TGF-beta1 differentiate naive $CD4^{+}CD25^{-}$ T cells into islet-protective Foxp3+ regulatory T cells. Proceedings of the National Academy of Sciences of the United States of America. 2007;**104**:2821-2826. DOI: 10.1073/pnas.0611646104

Chapter 5

Myelodysplastic Syndromes: An Update on Pathophysiology and Management

Wanxing Chai-Ho and Gary J. Schiller

Abstract

Myelodysplastic syndromes (MDS) comprise a set of clonal hematopoietic stem cell (HSC) disorders characterized by ineffective hematopoiesis that manifest as cytopenia of variable severity. The result often is an increased risk of infection, transfusion dependence, and a potential to transform to acute myeloid leukemia (AML). For the past decade, hypomethylating agents remain the only FDA-approved therapy. Given that MDS is more prevalent in the elderly who often have comorbid conditions, supportive care remains the mainstay of therapy. Curative treatments are restricted to younger, healthy individuals with histocompatible-matched donors for allogeneic transplant able to tolerate more intensive chemotherapeutic treatment. Understanding of the pathophysiology of MDS advanced over the past decade, which leads to an increasing array of new agents under clinical investigation. This review focuses on our recent enhanced understanding of MDS molecular biology, and promising novel agents that go beyond the hypomethylating agent.

Keywords: myelodysplastic syndrome (MDS), acute myeloid leukemia (AML), bone marrow transplant, hypomethylating agent, somatic mutation

1. Introduction

The myelodysplastic syndromes (MDS) comprise an heterogeneous group of malignant hematopoietic stem cell disorders characterized by dysplastic and ineffective blood cell production and a variable risk of transformation to acute leukemia. Based on the United States Surveillance, Epidemiology, and End Results (SEER) Program, the incidence of MDS is about 4.1–4.6 cases per 100,000 population per year, with approximately 86% of patients aged ≥60 years at time of diagnosis (median age 76 years). The incidence rate is higher in men than women. [1] The prevalence is slightly lower in Europe with reported 1.24–3.7 cases per 100,000 population per year, also with observed male predominance.[2, 3] With an aging population and improved awareness of disease, it is likely that the number of new patients diagnosed with MDS each year will increase in the future.

Pathogenesis of MDS is incompletely understood. Studies have revealed age, male gender, alcohol, cigarette smoking, ionizing radiation, chemotherapy such as alkylating agents and topoisomerase II inhibitor, immunosuppressive therapy, viral infection, benzene and other environmental/occupational exposures as possible implicating factors. [4–8] However, disease caused by these risk factors are estimated to account for only 20–30% of cases, which are described as secondary MDS, with remainders as primary MDS [4]. The major subsets of secondary MDS are therapy-related MDS (t-MDS) and MDS with predisposition to familial myeloid neoplasm.

The risk for MDS and AML is increased in certain familial predisposition syndromes, such as inherited bone marrow failure disorders like Diamond-Blackfan syndrome, Fanconi anemia, dyskeratosis congenital, Shwachman-Diamond syndrome, and Down syndrome, Noonan syndrome/Noonan syndrome-like disorders and neurofibromatosis [9]. Accurate diagnosis and recognition of these syndromic disorders allows opportunities to improve clinical care. Genetic counseling should be offered to family members of affected individual. One should avoid using heterozygous sibling as bone marrow transplant donor. Recently, a growing number of germline mutations including CEBPA, DDX41, ANKRD26, ETV6, GATA2, RUNX1 were identified to associate with familial thrombocytopenia and development of MDS and acute leukemia in up to 40% of patients [10, 11]. Special attention should be noted that many patients with familial MDS and acute leukemia predisposition syndromes develop disease in adulthood rather than childhood. To increase awareness of this entity of disease, myeloid neoplasm with above mentioned germline predisposition was incorporated into the updated WHO 2016 classification [12].

2. Diagnosis

2.1 Clinical presentation

MDS usually presents as cytopenia in one or more lineage. Fatigue, dyspnea on exertion, infection, easy bruising or bleeding are the most common symptoms. Lymphadenopathy and hepatosplenomegaly are infrequent and should raise suspicion for chronic myelomonocytic leukemia (CMML) [13, 14]. It has been estimated that various autoimmune features such as subacute vasculitis, fever, arthritis, peripheral edema, and pulmonary infiltrates, may be present in up to 10% of patients [15–18]. Certain autoimmune syndromes have correlated with distinct cytogenetic abnormalities; including Behcet's disease with trisomy 8, Sweet's syndrome and pyoderma gangrenosum with del(5q) [19]. Acquired hemoglobin H disease has been documented in approximately 8% of cases of MDS [20–22]. An acquired somatic mutation of ATRX, an X-linked gene encoding a chromatin-associated protein, has been linked to this entity, [21] as have acquired deletions of the alpha globin loci.

2.2 Pathology evaluation and WHO criteria

Bone marrow aspiration and biopsy are critical to the diagnosis of MDS. In general, the marrow is normo- or hypercellular due to ineffective hematopoiesis. However, up to 20% of MDS patients have hypocellular marrow, making it difficult to distinguish from aplastic anemia or paroxysmal nocturnal hematuria [23, 24]. Dysplastic neutrophils are commonly found in the peripheral blood smear. These cells may demonstrate reduced segmentation, increased size, the so-called pseudo-Pelger-Huet cell [25], often accompanied by reduced or absent granulation [26], and are associated with del(17)p [27]. Hypersegmentation with greater than 5 nuclear lobes is another feature of neutrophil dysplasia [28]. Red cells are usually normocytic or macrocytic, although ring sideroblasts, ovalomacrocytosis, teardrops, stomatocytes or acanthocytes may be seen [28]. Platelet morphology is usually normal, but micromegakaryocytes, mononuclear megakaryocytes, dumbbell-shaped nuclei, multinuclearity with multiple isolated nuclei ("Pawn ball" changes) may be seen [29].

Classification of MDS has been a challenge. In 1982, the French-American-British (FAB) Cooperative Group published the first seminal classification system that distinguished five subcategories of MDS based on marrow morphological criteria and myeloblasts proportions: refractory anemia, refractory anemia with ring sideroblasts (RARS), refractory anemia with excess of blasts (RAEB), RAEB "in transformation" (RAEB-T), and chronic myelomonocytic leukemia (CMML) [30]. Presence of more than 30% blasts in the bone marrow was defined as AML.

In 2001, World Health Organization (WHO) published new classification system on myeloid malignancy with modifications to the FAB system: The diagnosis of AML requires 20% myeloblasts. RAEB-T is classified as AML, and CMML is categorized as a new entity of myeloid neoplasms with both MDS and myeloproliferative features. In addition, MDS with isolated del(5q) is acknowledged as distinctive features in forms of disease with a low blast count, severe anemia and thrombocytosis (5q- syndrome) [31]. The revised 2008 WHO criteria maintained these modifications [32]. In the absence of definitive morphologic features of MDS, MDS-defining cytogenetic abnormalities were included in the diagnostic criteria (**Table 1**). The presence of chromosome 7, Y, or del(20q) does not meet criteria as an MDS-defining abnormality.

The 2016 revision of WHO (**Table 2**) incorporated rapidly accumulating molecular genetic information into the classification [12]. The same cytogenetic abnormalities listed in the 2008 WHO classification remain MDS-defining in a cytopenic patient. Given recent data showing 1 chromosomal abnormality in addition to the del(5q) poses no adverse effect [33–35], the entity "5q- syndrome" may be diagnosed if there is 1 additional cytogenetic abnormality besides the del(5q), unless that abnormality is monosomy 7 or del(7q). Mutations like SF3B1, TET2, SRSF2, ASXL1, DNMT3A, RUNX1, U2AF1, TP53, and EZH2 can be found in 80–90% MDS patients [36, 37]. Importantly, acquired clonal mutations identical to those seen in MDS can occur in the hematopoietic cells of healthy older individuals without MDS, so-called "clonal hematopoiesis of indeterminate potential" (CHIP), or patients with mild cytopenia but without dysplastic changes or specific cytogenetic and/or genetic abnormalities considered as presumptive evidence of MDS (idiopathic cytopenia of undetermined significance, ICUS) [38, 39]. Although some CHIP and ICUS subsequently develop MDS, there have not been sufficient data to support using the presence of aforementioned mutations as surrogate diagnostic marker of MDS. Based on the link between ring sideroblasts and an SF3B1 mutation, MDS

Unbalanced abnormalities	Balanced abnormalities
−7 or del(7q)	t(11;16)(q23;p13.3)
−5 or del(5q)	t(3;21)(q26.2;q22.1)
i(17q) or t(17p)	t(1;3)(p36.3;q21.1)
−13 or del(13q)	t(2;11)(p21;q23)
del(11q)	inv(3)(q21q26.2)
del(12p) or t(12p)	t(6;9)(p23;q34)
del(9q)	
idic(X)(q13)	
Complex karyotype (3 or more chromosomal abnormalities) involving one or more of the above abnormalities.	

Table 1.
Recurring chromosomal abnormalities considered as presumptive evidence of MDS in the setting of persistent cytopenia or undetermined origin in the absence of definitive morphologic features of MDS, according to World Health Organization 2008 and 2016 criteria.

Myeloproliferative neoplasms
Myeloid/lymphoid neoplasms with eosinophilia and rearrangement of PDGFRA, PDGFRB, or FGFR1, or with PCM1-JAK2
Myelodysplastic/myeloproliferative neoplasms (MDS/MPN) Chronic myelomonocytic leukemia(CMML) Atypical chronic myeloid leukemia (aCML), BCR-ABL1 Juvenile myelomonocytic leukemia (JMML) MDS/MPN with ring sideroblasts and thrombocytosis (MDS/MPN-RS-T) MDS/MPN, unclassifiable
Myelodysplastic syndrome MDS with single lineage dysplasia MDS with ring sideroblasts (MDS-RS) MDS-RS and single lineage dysplasia MDS-RS and multilineage dysplasia MDS with multilineage dysplasia MDS with excess blasts MDS with isolated del(5q) MDS, unclassifiable *Provisional entity: Refractory cytopenia of childhood*
Myeloid neoplasms with germline predisposition
Acute myeloid leukemia (AML) and related neoplasms Includes AML with myelodysplasia-related changes and therapy-related myeloid neoplasms
Blastic plasmacytoid dendritic cell neoplasm
Acute leukemias of ambiguous lineage
B-lymphoblastic leukemia/lymphoma
T-lymphoblastic leukemia/lymphoma

Table 2.
Classification of myeloid neoplasms and acute leukemia, according to World Health Organization 2016 criteria.

with ring sideroblasts and multilineage dysplasia, marked thrombocytosis, lacking excess blasts or an isolated del(5q) abnormality is included into the category of MDS with ring sideroblasts, and correlates with a favorable prognosis [40–43].

2.3 Differential diagnosis

MDS must be distinguished from other marrow dysplasia secondary to reversible causes, such as folate and vitamin B12 deficiency, viral infections (e.g. HIV), antibiotics, benzene, ethanol, or lead poisoning. Other primary bone marrow disorders presenting as pancytopenia, such as aplastic anemia, paroxysmal nocturnal hematuria, hairy cell leukemia, large granular lymphocytic leukemia can be distinguished by marrow morphology, flow cytometry features and gene mutation profile [8].

2.4 Risk stratification

The natural history of MDS in patients varies. The heterogeneity reflects both known and unknown differences in the pathophysiology of specific disease subtypes and patient related characteristics. Several prognostic scoring systems were developed and validated for MDS patients. In 1996, the International Prognostic Scoring System (IPSS) was developed by the International MDS Risk Analysis Workshop based on FAB classification [44]. Based on percent bone marrow blasts, specific cytogenetic abnormalities, and the number of cell lines involved with dysplasia and cytopenia, individual patient are placed into 4 groups: low, intermediate-1, intermediate-2, and high. The median survival in these four risk categories is 5.7 years for low risk, 3.5 years for intermediate-1 risk, 1.2 years for intermediate-2 risk, and 0.4 year for high risk.

In 2012, a revised IPSS (IPSS-R) was developed based upon data from 7012 patients with primary MDS diagnosed using the FAB or WHO classifications [45]. It incorporated new cytogenetic categories [35], and differentially weighed the degree of cytopenias in newly diagnosed patients. Patient age is an optional variable that can be incorporated to predict overall survival, but not evolution to AML. Individual patient was categorized into five risk groups: very low, low, intermediate, high and very high risk, that translates into median survival of 8.8, 5.3, 3.0, 1.6 and 0.8 years respectively. IPSS-R is simple to use, and is perhaps the most commonly used prognostication system today. However, there are several potential limitations to the IPSS-R. Both IPSS and IPSS-R were developed using data from patients who were observed without treatment. While outcomes might be different now that a variety of interventions are available, an analysis of a separate population suggested that the predictive value of the IPSS-R also applies to those treated with lenalidomide and azacitidine. [46] The prognosticating system only considered patients with *de novo* MDS. It is well recognized that patients with secondary MDS are more likely to have shorter survival. Much of this reflects the association between secondary MDS and "unfavorable cytogenetics". In addition, the IPSS-R seems to be most reliable at predicting outcomes at initial disease diagnosis, as the hazards in mortality and leukemia transformation diminishes over time in higher-risk but remains stable in lower-risk patients [47]. With increasing knowledge of MDS clonal genetics, the future risk stratification system might incorporate the prognostic value of mutation profile, which will be discussed in the next section.

WHO prognostic scoring system (WPSS) was designed to include information on red blood cell (RBC) transfusion need and cytogenetic information [48]. A subset of patients in the study cohort had data from multiple time points for a time-dependent analysis, therefore had the advantage over the IPSS of being able to be used at any time during the disease course.

The MD Anderson Cancer Center (MADCC) MDS model was developed based on a retrospective analysis of 856 patients with *de novo* or therapy-related MDS [49]. Age, cytogenetics, degree of anemia and thrombocytopenia, bone marrow blast percentage were identified as prognostic markers. Subsequently it was prospectively validated in 1915 patients, accounted for the duration of MDS and prior therapy [49]. One should take note that the MDACC model should only be applied to the population of patients with lower-risk (low or intermediate-1 IPSS) MDS, and patients who received various of MDS treatment, from which it was derived [50].

3. Pathogenesis

The pathogenesis of MDS is considered as a multistep process involving sequential acquisition of oncogenic mutations [51, 52]. The interplay between genetically altered HSCs and an abnormal bone marrow microenvironment may allow for selection of a predominant dysplastic clone [51–56].

3.1 Clonal heterogeneity and evolution

MDS is driven by a multistep process characterized by recurrent mutations affecting basic cellular pathways, including RNA splicing, epigenome regulation, myeloid transcription coordination, DNA damage response and growth factor signaling. It has been long recognized that HSC with certain pathogenic alterations has a competitive advantage and drives clonal expansion at the stem cell level. Clonal cytogenetic abnormalities are detected in up to 50% of *de novo* MDS cases and 80% of therapy-related cases [57, 58]. Over the past decade, a number of large, MDS-focused sequencing studies further demonstrated that MDS is a genetically complex and heterogeneous disease [36, 37, 42, 59–61].

However, clonality alone is not sufficient to cause or diagnose disease, because increased clonal hematopoiesis can remain functionally intact [38, 39]. Recently published data on a large cohort of cytopenia (ICUS) patients delineated the natural history of patients with clonal vs. nonclonal cytopenia [62]. Patients with clonal ICUS had a much higher rate of progression than patient with nonclonal ICUS. Spliceosome gene mutations such as SF3B1 SRSF2 and U2AF1 and co-mutation patterns involving TET2, DNMT3A or ASXL1 had clinical characteristics resemble low-risk MDS patients, and higher progression to myeloid neoplasm when comparing with patient with somatic TET2, DNMT3A and ASXL1 mutation alone [39].

The diversity of clinical MDS phenotypes associated with specific mutations may be related to differential coregulation of the HSC self-renewal and lineage-specific differentiation capacity. Accurate prediction of the natural history of individual patient is certainly of high clinic interest. Our growing knowledge suggests that individual mutations occur in highly stereotyped order and strong patterns of co-mutation association and exclusivity (**Figure 1**) [36, 60, 63]. Mutations affecting epigenetic modifier genes (DNMT3A, TET2, ASXL1, EZH2, etc.) or RNA spliceosome components (SF3B1, SRSF2, and U2AF1) tend to arise in the initiation and early progression phase of MDS and rarely occur at the time of transformation. By contrast, mutations in growth factor signaling pathways (NRAS, KRAS, PTPN11, FLT3, etc.) are rarely found in early phase of disease, and instead, they are frequently acquired and expanded in subclones at time of progression to high-grade MDS or secondary AML [63–66]. A recent study [67] suggested that at the time of

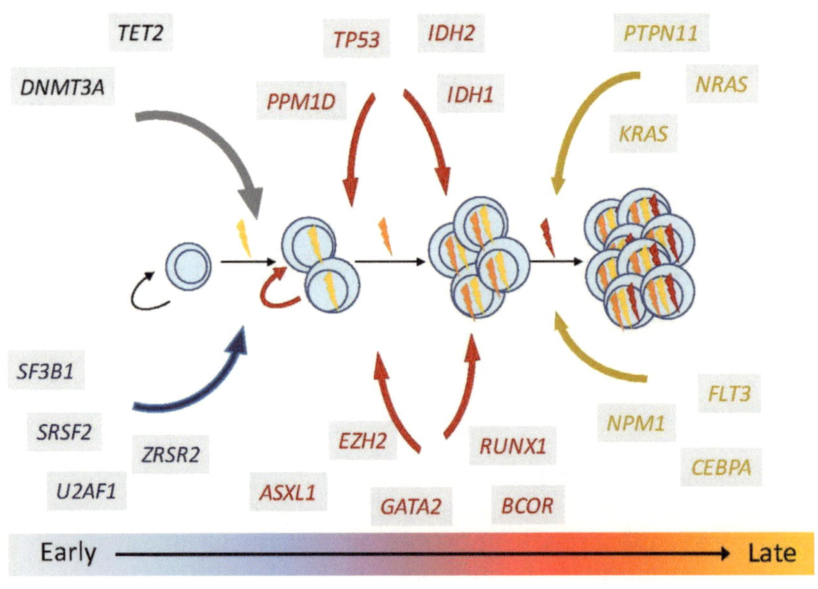

Figure 1.
Gene mutations have stereotyped positions in the MDS clonal hierarchy. Recent knowledge suggests that individual mutations occurs in highly stereotyped order and strong patterns of co-mutation association and exclusivity (Mutations affecting epigenetic modifier genes (DNMT3A, TET2, ASXL1, EZH2, etc.) or RNA spliceosome components (SF3B1, SRSF2, and U2AF1) tend to arise in the initiation and early progression phase of MDS and rarely occur at the time of transformation. Mutations in growth factor signaling pathways (NRAS, KRAS, PTPN11, FLT3, etc.) are frequently acquired and expanded in subclones at time of progression to high-grade MDS or secondary AML.

secondary AML transformation, the founding clone persisted at high variant allele fraction, but there was selective emergence and dominance of at least one genetically distinct subclone. In t-MDS, mutations in PPM1D or TP53 were present in 46% of patients, and they were the only gene mutations that were significantly associated with t-MDS [63, 68–71].

Various studies have also assessed the value of risk stratification based on MDS mutation profile [36, 42, 72]. TP53, ETV6, ASXL1, EZH2 and RUNX1 mutation confers adverse outcomes that are independent of IPSS risk assessment. SF3B1, which is frequently mutated in patients with ring sideroblasts, is associated with distinct and favorable clinical features [37, 38, 40].

3.2 Bone marrow microenvironment

HSC and genetically altered HSC all reside in a highly complex and dynamic cellular microenvironment in the bone marrow, that is composed of endothelial cells, multipotent mesenchymal stem cells, and sympathetic nerve fibers. There have been many *in vivo* studies demonstrated the concept of niche-induced disease initiation of MDS [73, 74] or AML [75, 76]. Evidence to support this in humans is mainly based on the not-so-rare occurrence of donor-derived leukemia in bone marrow transplant recipients, where changes in the preexisting niche in the host is thought to be leukemogenic [77]. In the review by Pleyer et al., [78] a variety of functional and molecular alterations were observed in *ex vivo* expanded mesenchymal stromal cells from MDS and AML patients, including their differentiation potential and HSC supportive activities, as well as chromosomal aberrations, transcriptional, and epigenetic changes. *In vivo* evidence also suggested that endothelial cells-specific gene alterations causes myeloproliferative disorders [79, 80].

3.3 Dysregulated immune pathways

Regulators of inflammation and innate immunity have always been thought to play an important role in pathogenesis of malignancies, but only until recent have the specific immune effectors and their cell-intrinsic functional roles in MDS stem cell biology been elucidated [81, 82]. Therapeutic targeting of over-activated innate immune components such as Toll-like receptors [83], IL-1 receptor–associated kinase/tumor necrosis factor receptor–associated factor-6 [84], IL8/CXCR2 [85], and IL1RAP [86] signaling pathways in MDS HSCs is being attempted pre-clinically.

4. Treatment

Treatment for MDS is guided by clinical symptoms, disease risk classification, patient age, comorbidities and performance status. Supportive care with transfusion and timely treatment of infection with antibiotics are important adjuncts for all MDS patients. Incorporating iron chelation therapy for patients requiring chronic transfusion and all candidates for allogeneic stem cell transplant is being increasingly emphasized to prevent cardiac and liver damage from iron overload [87, 88]. Pharmacologic treatment is usually reserved for symptomatic patients. Treatment goal for lower-risk MDS patients is to minimize symptoms, improve quality of life, and avoid toxicity from therapy. Erythropoiesis stimulating agent (ESA) can be used for symptomatic anemia and a low serum erythropoietin [89–92]. Together with low-dose G-CSF, hemoglobin improvement can be seen in up to 40% of lower-risk patients [93, 94]. Immunosuppressive therapy with anti-thymocyte globulin and cyclosporine A can produce response in a selected subset of patients. Those most likely to benefit are younger than 60 years, with less than 5% bone marrow blasts, hypoplastic MDS, presence of a paroxysmal nocturnal hemoglobinuria clone, trisomy 8, human leukocyte antigen DR15 positive, and with short duration of transfusion dependence [95]. Low-dose lenalidomide at 10 mg daily is FDA-approved for lower-risk MDS characterized as the 5q- syndrome. Transfusion independence was achieved in 67% of patients in the phase 2 trial [96], and 56% in the phase 3 trial [97]. For ESA refractory lower-risk MDS patients without 5q- syndrome, lenalidomide in combination with ESA also demonstrated efficacy at reducing transfusion need [98–100]. So far, the only FDA approved therapies for higher-risk MDS are the HMAs azacitidine and decitabine. The use of these agents results in complete (CR) and partial response (PR) each in 10–20% patients, with median duration of response about 10 months [101–104]. An additional 20–30% patients achieve hematologic improvement without an objective response. Despite survival benefit demonstrated with azacitidine in high-risk patients [101], HMAs are not curative. For young and fit patients, allogeneic stem cell transplant is the only curative treatment option. Therefore, there remains a significant unmet therapeutic need beyond HMAs. Novel agents under clinical investigation and the use of allogeneic stem cell transplant will be discussed here.

4.1 Next-generation hypomethylating agents

HMAs are S-phase specific. Conventional HMAs all have a very short half-lives (less than 30 min) due to rapid clearance of azanucleoside by cytidine deaminase. The focus of newer generation HMA development has been to meet the need of prolonged drug exposure, allowing greater drug incorporation into DNA.

Oral film-coated azacitidine (CC-486) was first studied in an open-label pilot trial. It demonstrated 17% mean bioavailability after a single dose at 80 mg [105]. In a subsequent phase 1 dose finding study in MDS, CMML and AML patients, overall response rate was 73% in previously untreated patients, and 35% in previously treated patients [106]. Extended dosing schedule of CC-486 for 14 or 21 days is being evaluated in a phase 3 trial (NCT01566695) in lower-risk MDS [107]. CC-486 is also being studied in combination with immune check point inhibitor in the second line setting (NCT02281084).

ASTX727 is a novel formulation of oral decitabine paired with an oral cytidine deaminase inhibitor E7727 to overcome the rapid clearance from cytidine deaminase in gut and liver. In the early phase studies with intermediate- or high-risk MDS, ASTX727 (35 mg decitabine, 100 mg E7227) successfully emulated the pharmacokinetic profile of intravenous decitabine [108, 109]. In the phase 2 trial, clinical benefit was observed in 62% patients, with 16% CR, 28% marrow complete response (mCR), and 18% hematologic improvement [109].

Another strategy to circumvent the rapid degradation of azanucleotide is to develop a novel formulation that is relatively resistant to cytidine deamination. Guadecitabine (SGI-110) is a novel dinucleotide of decitabine and deoxyguanosine, linked by a phosphodiester bond, that leads to a slower release of the active decitabine moiety, prolonging cellular exposure to the drug [110]. In the phase 2 study with guadecitabine in intermediate and high risk MDS and CMML patients, CR was observed in 7/49 treatment naïve patients (14%) while CR + mCR were observed in 11/53 previously treated patients (21%) [111].

4.2 Histone deacetylase inhibition

Both DNA-promoter hypomethylation as well as post-translational modification of histone tails (e.g., deacetylation) lead to transcriptional silencing of tumor-suppressor genes and genes involved in differentiation and apoptosis [112, 113]. Histone deacetylase inhibitors (HDACi) have limited single-agent efficacy in both high risk MDS and AML [114–116]. Preclinical evidence supported synergy between HMAs and HDACi [117]. However, a few phase 2 randomized clinical trials failed to demonstrate improvement in response rates or survival when azacitidine was combined with HDACi entinostat, vorinostat, valproic acid, or pracinostat [118–122]. Currently, a few clinical trials in MDS are ongoing using HDACi in combination with other novel agents such as immune checkpoint inhibitors (NCT 02936752) or pracinostat in combination with azacitidine using different dosing scheme (NCT 03151304). At this moment, how to best incorporate HDACi in MDS treatment remains uncertain.

4.3 Other epigenetic modification agents

Beyond targeting DNA methylation and HDAC recruitment, there has also been an increasing effort to develop epigenetic modification agents targeting posttranslation or posttranscription pathways, to mitigate malignant myeloid transformation in MDS.

Bromodomain and extraterminal (BET) proteins are epigenetic readers that recognize acetylated lysine tails of histones, and thus areas of open chromatin structure. It has been suggested that AML relies on BET protein BRD4 [123, 124], therefore led to great interest in utilizing BET inhibitors in myeloid malignancy. Various clinical trials are investigating the use of JQ1, the first selective BET inhibitor, in myeloid malignancy including MDS (NCT 02158858, NCT 02308761).

Overexpression of the mono and dimethyl lysine demethylase, LSD1 has been implicated in myeloid malignancies [125]. Clinical trials are ongoing evaluating LSD1 inhibitors in combination with ATRA or HMA in previously treated AML and MDS patients (NCT02273102, NCT02717884, NCT02929498).

4.4 Immune checkpoint inhibition

Upregulation of immune checkpoint molecules like PD-1/PDL-1 and CTLA4 is commonly observed in many malignancies, including AML and MDS [126, 127] to evade immune surveillance. However, preliminary experience suggested limited activity of immune checkpoint inhibitor use as single agent after HMA failure in MDS patients [128]. Several clinical trials are ongoing evaluating the efficacy of immune checkpoint inhibitors plus HMAs or HDACis (NCT02530463, NCT03092674, NCT02775903, NCT03094637, NCT02599649).

4.5 Other targeted therapies: extrapolating experience from AML

Based on the mutation profile, FLT3 inhibitor and IDH1/2 inhibitors are now FDA approved for AML. However, these mutations are less common in MDS [129]. The early phase ½ studies of IDH1 and IDH2 inhibitors included MDS patients, with reported response [130, 131]. Especially given their tolerability profile and single agent activity, these agents deserves further investigation in MDS.

Spliceosome mutations, such as SF3B1, SRSF2 and U2AF1 are the most common mutations in MDS [37]. Based on the encouraging activity in preclinical study [132], there is now a phase 1 study in myeloid malignancies including MDS, with splicing modulator H3B-8800, an oral modulator of the SF3B complex (NCT02841540).

Venetoclax, a selective BCL-2 inhibitor was granted breakthrough designation by FDA in combination with decitabine in 2017 for treatment–naive AML patients age greater than 65 years. This decision was based on result from two ongoing phase ½ clinical trials [133]. This combination is now being evaluated in higher-risk MDS in both frontline and HMA failure settings (NCT02966782, NCT02942290).

4.6 Management of anemia in lower-risk MDS

Luspatercept and sotatercept are modified activin receptor type II (ActRII) chimeric fusion proteins that consist of the modified extracellular domain of ActRIIB and ActRIIA respectively, trap TGF-β superfamily ligands to promote late-stage erythropoiesis [134, 135]. In the phase 2 trial of luspatercept for patients with lower-risk MDS who were ineligible for or refractory to ESAs, RBC transfusion independence was seen in 38% patients, and 63% hematologic improvement [136]. Similar efficacy was seen in the phase 2 trial for sotatercept, with 47% hematologic response in patients with high transfusion burden, and 58% with low transfusion burden [137]. Ongoing phase 3 clinical trial is evaluating the efficacy of ActRII antagonist in lower-risk MDS and MDS with ring sideroblasts who require regular RBC transfusions (NCT 02631070).

Rigosertib is a PI3K and polo-like kinase pathways small-molecule inhibitor. In the recent phase 2 study for transfusion-dependent lower-risk MDS patients, 20 of 62 (32%) patients achieved transfusion independence lasting for more than 8 weeks [138]. Validation of these results in future clinical trials is anticipated.

Roxadustat is a drug which acts as a HIF prolyl-hydroxylase inhibitor and thereby increases endogenous production of erythropoietin, which stimulates production of hemoglobin and RBCs. Roxadustat is shown to be safe and effective as anemia treatment for patient with underlying chronic kidney disease, not on dialysis [139]. A phase 3 trial is ongoing to evaluate the efficacy of roxadustat in low-risk MDS patients with low transfusion burden (NCT03263091).

4.7 Allogeneic stem cell transplant

Allogeneic stem cell transplant is the only curative therapy for MDS, but restricted to younger and fit patients. Disease free survival rates are approximately 30–50%. Treatment failure is attributed by transplant-related mortality in low-risk patients, and relapse in higher-risk patients [140]. In general, bone marrow transplant is offered to intermediate-2 and high-risk MDS patients. Over the past decade, reduced-intensity conditioning transplant made more older patients eligible for transplant [141]. An ongoing clinical trial is comparing the efficacy of reduced intensity allogeneic stem cell transplant to HMA in patients aged 50–75 with higher-risk disease [142]. In the study by Della Porta et al. [143], IPSS-R was prognostic for outcomes of patients in the high and very high-risk groups, but not in the low- and intermediate-risk groups.

There have been emerging data on the prognostic value of mutation profile and minimal residual disease pre- and post-transplantation. It was shown that only a minority of patients with MDS was in deep hematologic remission by flow cytometry minimal residual disease (MRD) and cytogenetic analysis before transplant [144]. For myeloablative conditioning, MRD positive and MRD negative patients had similar post-transplant outcome. However, relapse rate was higher for MRD positive patient who received non-myeloablative conditioning. Multiple studies have shown that TP53 mutation is an independent marker for short survival post-transplant [59, 61, 145]. EZH2, ETV6, RUNX1, ASXL1, JAK2, and mutations in the RAS signaling pathway have all been implicated to associate with short relapse-free interval post-transplant [59, 61, 145, 146].

5. Conclusion

Over the past decade, knowledge was gained in understanding the pathogenesis of MDS. However, many gaps remain to change the natural history of MDS. With increasing number of novel treatments under investigation, it is likely that we are getting closer to more therapeutics options for MDS in the near future.

Conflict of interest

Wanxing Chai-Ho reports no conflict-of-interest.

Gary Schiller receives research funding from Forma, Janssen, Onconova, Pfizer, Incyte and BioMed Valley Discoveries, and receives consulting fees from Agios, Amgen, Astellas, Bioline RX, Celgene, Gamida, Fanssen, Karyopharm, Leukemia Lymphoma Society, Medallion, Medeor, Merck, Pharmacyclics, Sanofi, Seattle Genetics, Spectrum, Stanford University Health, Sunesis, and Takeda.

Author details

Wanxing Chai-Ho and Gary J. Schiller*
UCLA Department of Medicine, Division of Hematology and Oncology, David Geffen School of Medicine, University of California, Los Angeles, CA, USA

*Address all correspondence to: gschiller@mednet.ucla.edu

References

[1] Ma X. Epidemiology of myelodysplastic syndromes. The American Journal of Medicine. 2012;**125**(7 Suppl):S2-S5. DOI: 10.1016/j.amjmed.2012.04.014

[2] Sant M, Allemani C, Tereanu C, et al. HAEMACARE Working GroupIncidence of hematologic malignancies in Europe by morphologic subtype: Results of the HAEMACARE project. Blood. 2010;**116**(19):3724-3734. DOI: 10.1182/blood-2010-05-282632

[3] Smith A, Howell D, Patmore R, et al. Incidence of haematological malignancy by sub-type: A report from the Haematological Malignancy Research Network. British Journal of Cancer. 2011;**105**(11):1684-1692. DOI: 10.1038/bjc.2011.450

[4] Finch SC. Myelodysplasia and radiation. Radiation Research. 2004;**161**:603-606

[5] Nisse C, Haguenoer JM, Grandbastien B, et al. Occupational and environmental risk factors of the myelodysplastic syndromes in the North of France. British Journal of Haematology. 2001;**112**:927-935

[6] Mundle S, Allampallam K, Rashid KA, et al. Presence of activation-related m-RNA for EBV and CMV in the bone marrow of patients with myelodysplastic syndromes. Cancer Letters. 2001;**164**:197-205

[7] Dalamaga M, Petridou E, Cook FE, et al. Risk factors for myelodysplastic syndromes: A case-control study in Greece. Cancer Causes & Control. 2002;**13**:603-608

[8] Catenacci DV, Schiller GJ. Myelodysplasic syndromes: A comprehensive review. Blood Reviews. 2005;**19**(6):301-319. DOI: 10.1016/j.blre.2005.01.004

[9] Owen C, Barnett M, Fitzgibbon J. Familial myelodysplasia and acute myeloid leukaemia—A review. British Journal of Haematology. 2008;**140**:123-132. DOI: 10.1111/j.1365-2141.2007.06909.x

[10] West AH, Godley LA, Churpek JE. Familial myelodysplastic syndrome/acute leukemia syndromes: A review and utility for translational investigations. Annals of the New York Academy of Sciences. 2014;**1310**:111-118. DOI: 10.1111/nyas.13543

[11] Babushok DV, Bessler M, Olson TS. Genetic predisposition to myelodysplastic syndrome and acute myeloid leukemia in children and young adults. Leukemia & Lymphoma. 2016;**57**(3):520-536. DOI: 10.3109/10428194.2015.1115041

[12] Arber DA, Orazi A, Hasserjian R, et al. The 2016 revision to the World Health Organization classification of myeloid neoplasms and acute leukemia. Blood. 2016;**127**(20):2391-2405. DOI: 10.1182/blood-2016-03-643544

[13] Cortes J. CMML: A biologically distinct myeloproliferative disease. Current Hematology Reports. 2003;**2**(3):202-208

[14] Bennett J. The myelodysplastic/myeloproliferative disorders: The interface. Hematology/Oncology Clinics of North America. 2003;**17**(5):1095-1100

[15] Enright H, Jacob H, Vercellotti G, et al. Paraneoplastic autoimmune phenomena in patients with myelodysplastic syndromes: Response to immunosuppressive therapy. British Journal of Haematology. 1995;**91**(2):403-408

[16] Saif MW, Hopkins JL, Gore SD. Autoimmune phenomena in patients

with myelodysplastic syndromes and chronic myelomonocytic leukemia. Leukemia and Lymphoma. 2002;**43**(11):2083-2092

[17] Giannouli M, Voulgarelis M, Zintzaras E, et al. Autoimmune phenomena in myelodysplastic syndromes: A 4-yr prospective study. Rheumatology. 2004;**43**:626-632. DOI: 10.1093/rheumatology/keh136

[18] Wolach O, Stone R. Autoimmunity and inflammation in myelodysplastic syndromes. Acta Haematologica. 2016;**136**(2):108. DOI: 10.1159/000446062

[19] Lee S, Park J, Lee E, et al. Certain autoimmune manifestations are associated with distinctive karyotypes and outcomes in patients with myelodysplastic syndrome: A retrospective cohort study. Medicine (Baltimore). 2016;**95**(13):e3091. DOI: 10.1097/MD.0000000000003091

[20] Steensma DP, Higgs DR, Fisher CA, et al. Acquired somatic ATRX mutations in myelodysplastic syndrome associated with alpha thalassemia (ATMDS) convey a more severe hematologic phenotype than germline ATRX mutations. Blood. 2004;**103**(6):2019. DOI: 10.1182/blood-2003-09-3360

[21] Steensma DP, Porcher JC, Hanson CA, et al. Prevalence of erythrocyte haemoglobin H inclusions in unselected patients with clonal myeloid disorders. British Journal of Haematology. 2007;**139**(3):439. DOI: 10.1111/j.1365-2141.2007.06831.x

[22] Higgs DR. Gene regulation in hematopoiesis: New lessons from thalassemia. Hematology. American Society of Hematology. Education Program. 2004;**2004**(1):1-13. DOI: 10.1182/asheducation-2004.1.1

[23] Wong KF, So CC. Hypoplastic myelodysplastic syndrome—A clinical, morphologic, or genetic diagnosis. Cancer Genetics and Cytogenetics. 2002;**138**:85-88

[24] Sloand EM. Hypocellular myelodysplasia. Hematology/Oncology Clinics of North America. 2009;**23**(2):347-360. DOI: 10.1016/j.hoc.2009.01.015

[25] Kuriyama K, Tomonaga M, Matsuo T, et al. Diagnostic significance of detecting pseudo-Pelger-Huët anomalies and micro-megakaryocytes in myelodysplastic syndrome. British Journal of Haematology. 1986;**63**(4):665

[26] Hast R, Nilsson I, Widell S, Ost A. Diagnostic significance of dysplastic features of peripheral blood polymorphs in myelodysplastic syndromes. Leukemia Research. 1989;**13**(2):173-178

[27] Soenen V, Preudhomme C, Roumier C, et al. 17p deletion in acute myeloid leukemia and myelodysplastic syndrome: Analysis of breakpoints and deleted segments by fluorescence in situ. Blood. 1998;**91**:1008-1015

[28] Giagounidis A, Haase D. Morphology, cytogenetics and classification of MDS. Best Practice & Research. Clinical Haematology. 2013;**26**(4):337-353. DOI: 10.1016/j.beha.2013.09.004

[29] Wong KF, Chan JK. Are 'dysplastic' and hypogranular megakaryocytes specific markers for myelodysplastic syndrome? British Journal of Haematology. 1991;**77**(4):509

[30] Bennett JM, Catovsky D, Daniel MT, et al. Proposals for the classification of the myelodysplastic syndromes. British Journal of Haematology. 1982;**51**:189-199

[31] Vardiman JW, Brunning RD, Harris NL. The World Health Organization (WHO) classification of the myeloid neoplasms. Blood.

2002;**100**(7):2292-2302. DOI: 10.1182/blood-2002-04-1199

[32] Vardiman JW, Thiele J, Arber DA, et al. The 2008 revision of the World Health Organization classification of myeloid neoplasms and acute leukemia: Rationale and important changes. Blood. 2009;**114**:937-951. DOI: 10.1182/blood-2009-03-209262

[33] Germing U, Lauseker M, Hildebrandt B, et al. Survival, prognostic factors and rates of leukemic transformation in 381 untreated patients with MDS and del(5q): A multicenter study. Leukemia. 2012;**26**(6):1286-1292. DOI: 10.1038/leu.2011.391

[34] Mallo M, Cervera J, Schanz J, et al. Impact of adjunct cytogenetic abnormalities for prognostic stratification in patients with myelodysplastic syndrome and deletion 5q. Leukemia. 2011;**25**(1):110-120. DOI: 10.1038/leu.2010.231

[35] Schanz J, Tüchler H, Solé F, et al. New comprehensive cytogenetic scoring system for primary myelodysplastic syndromes (MDS) and oligoblastic acute myeloid leukemia after MDS derived from an international database merge. Journal of Clinical Oncology. 2012;**30**(8):820-829. DOI: 10.1200/JCO.2011.35.6394

[36] Papaemmanuil E, Gerstung M, Malcovati L, et al. Clinical and biological implications of driver mutations in myelodysplastic syndromes. Blood. 2013;**122**(22):3616-3627. DOI: 10.1182/blood-2013-08-518886

[37] Haferlach T, Nagata Y, Grossmann V, et al. Landscape of genetic lesions in 944 patients with myelodysplastic syndromes. Leukemia. 2014;**28**(2):241-247. DOI: 10.1038/leu.2013.336

[38] Jaiswal S, Fontanillas P, Flannick J, et al. Age-related clonal hematopoiesis associated with adverse outcomes. The New England Journal of Medicine. 2014;**371**(26):2488-2498. DOI: 10.1056/NEJMoa1408617

[39] Genovese G, Kähler AK, Handsaker RE, et al. Clonal hematopoiesis and blood-cancer risk inferred from blood DNA sequence. The New England Journal of Medicine. 2014;**371**(26):2477-2487. DOI: 10.1056/NEJMoa1409405

[40] Malcovati L, Papaemmanuil E, Bowen DT, et al. Clinical significance of SF3B1 mutations in myelodysplastic syndromes and myelodysplastic/myeloproliferative neoplasms. Blood. 2011;**118**(24):6239-6246. DOI: 10.1182/blood-2011-09-377275

[41] Papaemmanuil E, Cazzola M, Boultwood J, et al. Somatic SF3B1 mutation in myelodysplasia with ring sideroblasts. The New England Journal of Medicine. 2011;**365**(15):1384-1395. DOI: 10.1056/NEJMoa1103283

[42] Bejar R, Stevenson KE, Caughey BA, et al. Validation of a prognostic model and the impact of mutations in patients with lower-risk myelodysplastic syndromes. Journal of Clinical Oncology. 2012;**30**(27):3376-3382. DOI: 10.1200/JCO.2011.40.7379

[43] Cazzola M, Rossi M, Malcovati L, et al. Biologic and clinical significance of somatic mutations of SF3B1 in myeloid and lymphoid neoplasms. Blood. 2013;**121**(2):260-269. DOI: 10.1182/blood-2012-09-399725

[44] Greenberg P, Cox C, LeBeau MM, et al. International scoring system for evaluating prognosis in myelodysplastic syndromes. Blood. 1997;**89**(6):2079-2088

[45] Greenberg PL, Tuechler H, Schanz J, et al. Revised international prognostic scoring system for myelodysplastic syndromes. Blood. 2012;**120**(12):2454. DOI: 10.1182/blood-2012-03-420489

[46] Voso MT, Fenu S, Latagliata R, et al. Revised international prognostic scoring system (IPSS) predicts survival and leukemic evolution of myelodysplastic syndromes significantly better than IPSS and WHO prognostic scoring system: Validation by the Gruppo Romano Mielodisplasie Italian Regional Database. Journal of Clinical Oncology. 2013;**31**(21):2671. DOI: 10.1200/JCO.2012.48.0764

[47] Pfeilstöcker M, Tuechler H, Sanz G, et al. Time-dependent changes in mortality and transformation risk in MDS. Blood. 2016;**128**(7):902-910. DOI: 10.1182/blood-2016-02-700054

[48] Malcovati L, Germing U, Kuendgen A, et al. Time-dependent prognostic scoring system for predicting survival and leukemic evolution in myelodysplastic syndromes. Journal of Clinical Oncology. 2007;**25**(23):3503-3510. DOI: 10.1200/JCO.2006.08.5696

[49] Kantarjian H, O'Brien S, Ravandi F, et al. Proposal for a new risk model in myelodysplastic syndrome that accounts for events not considered in the original international prognostic scoring system. Cancer. 2008;**113**(6):1351-1361. DOI: 10.1002/cncr.23697

[50] Garcia-Manero G, Shan J, Faderl S, et al. A prognostic score for patients with lower risk myelodysplastic syndrome. Leukemia. 2008;**22**(3):538-543. DOI: 10.1038/sj.leu.2405070

[51] Warlick ED, Smith BD. Myelodysplastic syndromes: Review of pathophysiology and current novel treatment approaches. Current Cancer Drug Targets. 2007;7:541-558

[52] Fenaux P. Myelodysplastic syndromes: From pathogenesis and prognosis to treatment. Seminars in Hematology. 2004;**41**(2 Suppl. 4):13-20

[53] Lindsley RC. Uncoding the genetic heterogeneity of myelodysplastic syndrome. Hematology. American Society of Hematology. Education Program. 2017;**2017**(1):447-452. DOI: 10.1182/asheducation-2017.1.447

[54] Shastri A, Will B, Steidl U, Verma A. Stem and progenitor cell alterations in myelodysplastic syndromes. Blood. 2017;**129**(12):1586-1594. DOI: 10.1182/blood-2016-10-696062

[55] Li AJ, Calvi LM. The microenvironment in myelodysplastic syndromes: Niche-mediated disease initiation and progression. Experimental Hematology. 2017;**55**:3-18. DOI: 10.1016/j.exphem.2017.08.003

[56] Medyouf H. The microenvironment in human myeloid malignancies: Emerging concepts and therapeutic implications. Blood. 2017;**129**(12):1617-1626. DOI: 10.1182/blood-2016-11-696070

[57] Maurtizson N, Albin N, Rylander L, et al. Pooled analysis of clinical and cytogenetic features in treatment-related and de novo adult acute myloid leukemia and myelodysplastic syndromes based on a consecutive series of 761 patients analyzed 1976-1993 and on 5098 unselected cases reported in the literature 1974-2001. Leukemia. 2002;**16**(12):2366-2378. DOI: 10.1038/sj.leu.2402713

[58] Olney HJ, LeBeau MM. The cytogenetics of myelodysplastic syndromes. Best Practice & Research Clinical Haematology. 2001;**14**(3):479-495. DOI: 10.1053/beha.2001.0151

[59] Lindsley RC, Saber W, Mar BG, et al. Prognostic mutations in myelodysplastic syndrome after stem-cell transplantation. The New England Journal of Medicine. 2017;**376**(6):536-547. DOI: 10.1056/NEJMoa1611604

[60] Makishima H, Yoshizato T, Yoshida K, et al. Dynamics of clonal evolution in myelodysplastic syndromes.

Nature Genetics. 2017;**49**(2):204-212. DOI: 10.1038/ng.3742

[61] Yoshizato T, Nannya Y, Atsuta Y, et al. Genetic abnormalities in myelodysplasia and secondary acute myeloid leukemia: Impact on outcome of stem cell transplantation. Blood. 2017;**129**(17):2347-2358. DOI: 10.1182/blood-2016-12-754796

[62] Malcovati L, Gallì A, Travaglino E, et al. Clinical significance of somatic mutation in unexplained blood cytopenia. Blood. 2017;**129**(25):3371-3378. DOI: 10.1182/blood-2017-01-763425

[63] Lindsley RC, Mar BG, Mazzola E, et al. Acute myeloid leukemia ontogeny is defined by distinct somatic mutations. Blood. 2015;**125**(9):1367-1376. DOI: 10.1182/blood-2014-11-610543

[64] Corces-Zimmerman MR, Hong W-J, Weissman IL, Medeiros BC, Majeti R. Preleukemic mutations in human acute myeloid leukemia affect epigenetic regulators and persist in remission. Proceedings of the National Academy of Sciences of the United States of America. 2014;**111**(7):2548-2553. DOI: 10.1073/pnas.1324297111

[65] Badar T, Patel KP, Thompson PA, et al. Detectable FLT3-ITD or RAS mutation at the time of transformation from MDS to AML predicts for very poor outcomes. Leukemia Research. 2015;**39**(12):1367-1374. DOI: 10.1016/j.leukres.2015.10.005

[66] Kim T, Tyndel MS, Kim HJ, et al. The clonal origins of leukemic progression of myelodysplasia. Leukemia. 2017;**31**(9):1928-1935. DOI: 10.1038/leu.2017.17

[67] Walter MJ, Shen D, Ding L, et al. Clonal architecture of secondary acute myeloid leukemia. The New England Journal of Medicine. 2012;**366**(12):1090-1098. DOI: 10.1056/NEJMoa1106968

[68] Takahashi K, Wang F, Kantarjian H, et al. Preleukaemic clonal haemopoiesis and risk of therapy-related myeloid neoplasms: A case-control study. The Lancet Oncology. 2017;**18**(1):100-111. DOI: 10.1016/S1470-2045(16)30626-X

[69] Wong TN, Ramsingh G, Young AL, et al. Role of TP53 mutations in the origin and evolution of therapy-related acute myeloid leukaemia. Nature. 2015;**518**(7540):552-555. DOI: 10.1038/nature13968

[70] Ok CY, Patel KP, Garcia-Manero G, et al. Mutational profiling of therapy-related myelodysplastic syndromes and acute myeloid leukemia by next generation sequencing, a comparison with de novo diseases. Leukemia Research. 2015;**39**(3):348-354. DOI: 10.1016/j.leukres.2014.12.006

[71] Shih AH, Chung SS, Dolezal EK, et al. Mutational analysis of therapy-related myelodysplastic syndromes and acute myelogenous leukemia. Haematologica. 2013;**98**(6):908-912. DOI: 10.3324/haematol.2012.076729

[72] Cargo CA, Rowbotham N, Evans PA, et al. Targeted sequencing identifies patients with preclinical MDS at high risk of disease progression. Blood. 2015;**126**(21):2362-2365. DOI: 10.1182/blood-2015-08-663237

[73] Schepers K, Campbell TB, Passegue E. Normal and leukemic stem cell niches: Insights and therapeutic opportunities. Cell Stem Cell. 2015;**16**(3):254-267. DOI: 10.1016/j.stem.2015.02.014

[74] Wiseman DH. Donor cell leukemia: A review. Biology of Blood and Marrow Transplantation. 2011;**17**(6):771-789. DOI: 10.1016/j.bbmt.2010.10.010

[75] Blau O, Baldus CD, Hofmann WK, et al. Mesenchymal stromal cells

of myelodysplastic syndrome and acute myeloid leukemia patients have distinct genetic abnormalities compared with leukemic blasts. Blood. 2011;**118**(20):5583-5592. DOI: 10.1182/blood-2011-03-343467

[76] Blau O, Hofmann WK, Baldus CD, et al. Chromosomal aberrations in bone marrow mesenchymal stroma cells from patients with myelodysplastic syndrome and acute myeloblastic leukemia. Experimental Hematology. 2007;**35**(2):221-229. DOI: 10.1016/j.exphem.2006.10.012

[77] Huang JC, Basu SK, Zhao X, et al. Mesenchymal stromal cells derived from acute myeloid leukemia bone marrow exhibit aberrant cytogenetics and cytokine elaboration. Blood Cancer Journal. 2015;**5**:e302. DOI: 10.1038/bcj.2015.17

[78] Pleyer L, Valent P, Greil R. Mesenchymal stem and progenitor cells in normal and dysplastic hematopoies is masters of survival and clonality? International Journal of Molecular Sciences. 2016;**17**(7):1009. DOI: 10.3390/ijms17071009

[79] Peled A, Petit I, Kollet O, et al. Dependence of human stem cell engraftment and repopulation of NOD/SCID mice on CXCR4. Science. 1999;**283**(5403):845-848

[80] Foster K, Lassailly F, Anjos-Afonso F, et al. Different motile behaviors of human hematopoietic stem versus progenitor cells at the osteoblastic niche. Stem Cell Reports. 2015;**5**(5):690-701. DOI: 10.1016/j.stemcr.2015.09.003

[81] Chen X, Eksioglu EA, Zhou J, et al. Induction of myelodysplasia by myeloid-derived suppressor cells. The Journal of Clinical Investigation. 2013;**123**(11):4595-4611. DOI: 10.1172/JCI67580

[82] Verma A, List AF. Cytokine targets in the treatment of myelodysplastic syndromes. Current Hematology Reports. 2005;**4**(6):429-435

[83] Varney ME, Melgar K, Niederkorn M, et al. Deconstructing innate immune signaling in myelodysplastic syndromes. Experimental Hematology. 2015;**43**(8):587-598. DOI: 10.1016/j.exphem.2015.05.016

[84] Gañán-Gómez I, Wei Y, Starczynowski DT, et al. Deregulation of innate immune and inflammatory signaling in myelodysplastic syndromes. Leukemia. 2015;**29**(7):1458-1469. DOI: 10.1038/leu.2015.69

[85] Schinke C, Giricz O, Li W, et al. IL8-CXCR2 pathway inhibition as a therapeutic strategy against MDS and AML stem cells. Blood. 2015;**125**(20):3144-3152. DOI: 10.1182/blood-2013-03-492884

[86] Ågerstam H, Hansen N, von Palffy S, et al. IL1RAP antibodies block IL-1-induced expansion of candidate CML stem cells and mediate cell killing in xenograft models. Blood. 2016;**128**(23):2683-2693. DOI: 10.1182/blood-2015-01-621631

[87] Malcovati L, Hellström-Lindberg E, Bowen D, et al. Diagnosis and treatment of primary myelodysplastic syndromes in adults: Recommendations from the European LeukemiaNet. Blood. 2013;**22**:2943-2964. DOI: 10.1182/blood-2013-03-492884

[88] NCCN (National Comprehensive Cancer Network). NCCN Clinical Practice Guidelines in Oncology: Myelodysplastic Syndromes. Version 1. 2019. Available from: https://www.nccn.org/professionals/physician_gls/pdf/mds.pdf [Accessed: 2016-10-12]

[89] Stenke L, Wallvik J, Celsing F, et al. Prediction of response to treatment with

human recombinant erythropoietin in myelodysplastic syndromes. Leukemia. 1993;7:1324-1327

[90] Stasi R, Brunetti M, Bussa S, et al. Response to recombinant human erythropoietin in patients with myelodysplastic syndromes. Clinical Cancer Research. 1997;**3**:733-739

[91] Rossi Ferrini PR, Grossi A, Vannucchi AM, et al. A randomized double-blind placebo-controlled study with subcutaneous recombinant human erythropoietin in patients with low-risk myelodysplastic syndromes. British Journal of Haematology. 1998;**103**:1070-1074

[92] Terpos E, Mougiou A, Kouraklis A, et al. Prolonged administration of erythropoietin increases erythroid response rate in myelodysplastic syndromes: A phase II trial in 281 patients. British Journal of Haematology. 2002;**118**:174-180

[93] Greenberg PL, Sun Z, Miller KB, et al. Treatment of myelodysplastic syndrome patients with erythropoietin with or without granulocyte colony-stimulating factor: Results of a prospective randomized phase 3 trial by the Eastern Cooperative Oncology Group (E1996). Blood. 2009;**114**(12):2393. DOI: 10.1182/blood-2009-03-211797

[94] Mantovani L, Lentini G, Hentschel B, et al. Treatment of anaemia in myelodysplastic syndromes with prolonged administration of recombinant human granulocyte colony-stimulating factor and erythropoietin. British Journal of Haematology. 2000;**109**(2):367

[95] Sloand EM, Wu CO, Greenberg P, et al. Factors affecting response and survival in patients with myelodysplasia treated with immunosuppressive therapy. Journal of Clinical Oncology. 2008;**26**(15):2505. DOI: 10.1200/JCO.2007.11.9214

[96] List A, Dewald G, Bennett J, et al. Lenalidomide in the myelodysplastic syndrome with chromosome 5q deletion. The New England Journal of Medicine. 2006;**355**(14):1456. DOI: 10.1056/NEJMoa061292

[97] Fenaux P, Giagounidis A, Selleslag D, et al. A randomized phase 3 study of lenalidomide versus placebo in RBC transfusion-dependent patients with low-/intermediate-1-risk myelodysplastic syndromes with del5q. Blood. 2011;**118**(14):3765. DOI: 10.1182/blood-2011-01-330126

[98] Komrokji RS, Lancet JE, Swern AS, et al. Combined treatment with lenalidomide and epoetin alfa in lower-risk patients with myelodysplastic syndrome. Blood. 2012;**120**:3419-3424. DOI: 10.1182/blood-2012-03-415661

[99] Sibon D, Cannas G, Baracco F, et al. Lenalidomide in lower-risk myelodysplastic syndromes with karyotypes other than deletion 5q and refractory to erythropoiesis-stimulating agents. British Journal of Haematology. 2012;**156**:619-625. DOI: 10.1111/j.1365-2141.2011.08979.x

[100] Toma A, Kosmider O, Chevret S, et al. Lenalidomide with or without erythropoietin in transfusion dependent erythropoiesis-stimulating agent-refractory lower risk MDS without 5qdeletion. Leukemia. 2016;**30**:897-905. DOI: 10.1038/leu.2015.296

[101] Fenaux P, Mufti GJ, Hellstrom-Lindberg E, et al. Efficacy of azacitidine compared with that of conventional care regimens in the treatment of higher-risk myelodysplastic syndromes: A randomised, open-label, phase III study. The Lancet Oncology. 2009;**10**(3):223-232. DOI: 10.1016/S1470-2045(09)70003-8

[102] Silverman LR, Fenaux P, Mufti GJ, et al. Continued azacitidine therapy beyond time of first response improves

quality of response in patients with higher-risk myelodysplastic syndromes. Cancer. 2011;**117**(12):2697-2702. DOI: 10.1002/cncr.25774

[103] Kantarjian H, Issa JP, Rosenfeld CS, et al. Decitabine improves patient outcomes in myelodysplastic syndromes: Results of a phase III randomized study. Cancer. 2006;**106**(8):1794-1803. DOI: 10.1002/cncr.21792

[104] Steensma DP, Baer MR, Slack JL, et al. Multicenter study of decitabine administered daily for 5 days every 4 weeks to adults with myelodysplastic syndromes: The alternative dosing for outpatient treatment (ADOPT) trial. Journal of Clinical Oncology. 2009;**27**(23):3842-3848. DOI: 10.1200/JCO.2008.19.6550

[105] Garcia-Manero G, Stoltz ML, Ward MR, et al. A pilot pharmacokinetic study of oral azacitidine. Leukemia. 2008;**22**(9):1680-1684. DOI: 10.1038/leu.2008.145

[106] Garcia-Manero G, Gore SD, Cogle C, et al. Phase I study of oral azacitidine in myelodysplastic syndromes, chronic myelomonocytic leukemia, and acute myeloid leukemia. Journal of Clinical Oncology. 2011;**29**(18):2521-2527. DOI: 10.1200/JCO.2010.34.4226

[107] Garcia-Manero G, Gore SD, Kambhampati S, et al. Efficacy and safety of extended dosing schedules of CC-486 (oral azacitidine) in patients with lower-risk myelodysplastic syndromes. Leukemia. 2016;**30**(4):889-896. DOI: 10.1038/leu.2015.265

[108] Garcia-Manero G, Odenike O, Amrin PC, et al. Successful emulation of IV decitabine pharmacokinetics with an oral fixed-dose combination of the oral cytidine deaminase inhibitor (CDAi) E7727 with oral decitabine, in subjects with myelodysplastic syndromes (MDS): Final data of phase 1 study. In the 58th American Society of Hematology annual meeting and exposition, 3-6 December 2016, San Diego, CA. Blood. 2016;**128**(22):114

[109] Garcia-Manero G, Griffiths EA, Roboz GJ, et al. A phase 2 dose-confirmation study of oral ASTX727, a combination of oral decitabine with a cytidine deaminase inhibitor (CDAi) cedazuridine (E7727), in subjects with myelodysplastic syndromes (MDS). In the 59th American Society of Hematology annual meeting and exposition, 9-12 December 2017, Atlanta, GA. Blood. 2017;**130**:4274

[110] Issa JJ, Roboz G, Rizzieri D, et al. Safety and tolerability of guadecitabine (SGI-110) in patients with myelodysplastic syndrome and acute myeloid leukaemia: A multicentre, randomised, dose-escalation phase 1 study. The Lancet Oncology. 2015;**16**(9):1099-1110. DOI: 10.1016/S1470-2045(15)00038-8

[111] Garcia-Manero GRE, Walsh K, et al. First clinical results of a randomized phase 2 dose-response study of SGI-110, a novel subcutaneous (SC) hypomethylating agent (HMA), in 102 patients with intermediate (int) or high risk (HR) myelodysplastic syndromes (MDS) or chronic myelomonocytic leukemia (CMML). In the 56th American Society of Hematology annual meeting and exposition, 6-9 December 2014, San Francisco, CA. Blood. 2014;**124**(21):529

[112] Herman JG, Baylin SB. Gene silencing in cancer in association with promoter hypermethylation. The New England Journal of Medicine. 2003;**349**(21):2042-2054. DOI: 10.1056/NEJMra023075

[113] Stahl M, Kohrman N, Gore SD, et al. Epigenetics in cancer: A hematological perspective. PLoS Genetics. 2016;**12**:e1006193. DOI: 10.1371/journal.pgen.1006193

[114] Stahl M, Gore SD, Vey N, Prebet T. Lost in translation? Ten years of development of histone deacetylase inhibitors in acute myeloid leukemia and myelodysplastic syndromes. Expert Opinion on Investigational Drugs. 2016;**25**:307-317. DOI: 10.1517/13543784.2016.1146251

[115] Schaefer EW, Loaiza-Bonilla A, Juckett M, et al. A phase 2 study of vorinostat in acute myeloid leukemia. Haematologica. 2009;**94**:1375-1382. DOI: 10.3324/haematol.2009.009217

[116] DeAngelo DJ, Spencer A, Bhalla KN, et al. Phase Ia/II, 2-arm, open-label, dose-escalation study of oral panobinostat administered via 2 dosing schedules in patients with advanced hematologic malignancies. Leukemia. 2013;**27**:1628-1636. DOI: 10.1038/leu.2013.38

[117] Cameron EE, Bachman KE, Myöhänen S, et al. Synergy of demethylation and histone deacetylase inhibition in the re-expression of genes silenced in cancer. Nature Genetics. 1999;**21**(1):103-107

[118] Tan P, Wei A, Mithraprabhu S, et al. Dual epigenetic targeting with panobinostat and azacitidine in acute myeloid leukemia and high risk myelodysplastic syndrome. Blood Cancer Journal. 2014;**4**:e170. DOI: 10.1038/bcj.2013.68

[119] Prebet T, Sun Z, Figueroa ME, et al. Prolonged administration of azacitidine with or without entinostat for myelodysplastic syndrome and acute myeloid leukemia with myelodysplasia-related changes: Results of the US leukemia intergroup trial E1905. Journal of Clinical Oncology. 2014;**32**:1242-1248. DOI: 10.1200/JCO.2013.50.3102

[120] Mikkael A, Sekeres MO, List AF, et al. Additional analyses of a randomized phase II study of azacitidine combined with lenalidomide or with vorinostat vs. azacitidine monotherapy in higher-risk myelodysplastic syndromes (MDS) and chronic myelomonocytic leukemia (CMML): North American intergroup study SWOG S1117. In the 57th American Society of Hematology annual meeting and exposition, 5-8 December 2015, Orlando, FL. Blood. 2015;**126**:908

[121] Issa JP, Garcia-Manero G, Huang X, et al. Results of phase 2 randomized study of low-dose decitabine with or without valproic acid in patients with myelodysplastic syndrome and acute myelogenous leukemia. Cancer. 2015;**121**:556-561. DOI: 10.1002/cncr.29085

[122] Garcia-Manero G, Montalban-Bravo G, Berdeja JG, et al. Phase 2, randomized, double-blind study of pracinostat in combination with azacitidine in patients with untreated, higher-risk myelodysplastic syndromes. Cancer. 2017;**123**(6):994-1002. DOI: 10.1002/cncr.30533

[123] Dawson MA, Prinjha RK, Dittmann A, et al. Inhibition of BET recruitment to chromatin as an effective treatment for MLL-fusion leukaemia. Nature. 2011;**478**(7370):529-533. DOI: 10.1038/nature10509

[124] Zuber J, Shi J, Wang E, et al. RNAi screen identifies Brd4 as a therapeutic target in acute myeloid leukaemia. Nature. 2011;**478**(7370):524-528. DOI: 10.1038/nature10334

[125] Schenk T, Chen WC, Göllner S, et al. Inhibition of the LSD1 (KDM1A) demethylase reactivates the all-trans-retinoic acid differentiation pathway in acute myeloid leukemia. Nature Medicine. 2012;**18**(4):605-611. DOI: 10.1038/nm.2661

[126] Zhang L, Gajewski TF, Kline J. PD-1/PD-L1 interactions inhibit antitumor immune responses in a murine acute myeloid leukemia model.

Blood. 2009;**114**(8):1545-1552. DOI: 10.1182/blood-2009-03-206672

[127] Yang H, Bueso-Ramos C, DiNardo C, et al. Expression of PD-L1, PD-L2, PD-1 and CTLA4 in myelodysplastic syndromes is enhanced by treatment with hypomethylating agents. Leukemia. 2014;**28**(6):1280-1288. DOI: 10.1038/leu.2013.355

[128] Garcia-Manero G, Daver N, Montalban-Bravo G, et al. A phase II study evaluating the combination of nivolumab (Nivo) or ipilimumab (Ipi) with azacitidine in pts with previously treated or untreated myelodysplastic syndromes (MDS). In the 58th american Society of Hematology annual meeting and exposition, 3-6 December 2016, San Diego, CA. Blood. 2016;**128**(22):344

[129] DiNardo CD, Jabbour E, Ravandi F, et al. IDH1 and IDH2 mutations in myelodysplastic syndromes and role in disease progression. Leukemia. 2016;**30**(4):980-984. DOI: 10.1038/leu.2015.211

[130] Stein EM, DiNardo CD, Pollyea DA, et al. Enasidenib in mutant IDH2 relapsed or refractory acute myeloid leukemia. Blood. 2017;**130**(6):722-731. DOI: 10.1182/blood-2017-04-779405

[131] CD DN, de Botton S, Stein EM, et al. Determination of IDH1 mutational burden and clearance via next-generation sequencing in patients with IDH1 mutation-positive hematologic malignancies receiving AG-120, a first-in-class inhibitor of mutant IDH1. In the 58th american Society of Hematology annual meeting and exposition, 3-6 December 2016, San Diego, CA. Blood. 2016;**128**(22):1070

[132] Buonamici SY, Yoshimi A, Thomas M, et al. H3B-8800, an orally bioavailable modulator of the SF3b complex, shows efficacy in spliceosome-mutant myeloid malignancies. In the 58th American Society of Hematology annual meeting and exposition, 3-6 December 2016, San Diego, CA. Blood. 2016;**128**(22):966

[133] DiNardo C, Pollyea DA, Pratz K, et al. A phase 1b study of venetoclax (ABT-199/GDC-0199) in combination with decitabine or azacitidine in treatment-naive patients with acute myelogenous leukemia who are ≥ to 65 years and not eligible for standard induction therapy. In the 58th American Society of Hematology annual meeting and exposition, 3-6 December 2016, San Diego, CA. Blood. 2015;**126**:327

[134] Suragani RN, Cadena SM, Cawley SM, et al. Transforming growth factor-β superfamily ligand trap ACE-536 corrects anemia by promoting late-stage erythropoiesis. Nature Medicine. 2014;**20**(4):408-414. DOI: 10.1038/nm.3512

[135] Dussiot M, Maciel TT, Fricot A, et al. An activin receptor IIA ligand trap corrects ineffective erythropoiesis in β-thalassemia. Nature Medicine. 2014;**20**(4):398-407. DOI: 10.1038/nm.3468

[136] Platzbecker U, Germing U, Götze KS, et al. Luspatercept for the treatment of anaemia in patients with lower-risk myelodysplastic syndromes (PACE-MDS): A multicentre, open-label phase 2 dose-finding study with long-term extension study. The Lancet Oncology. 2017;**18**(10):1338-1347. DOI: 10.1016/S1470-2045(17)30615-0

[137] Komrokji R, Garcia-Manero G, Ades L, et al. Sotatercept with long-term extension for the treatment of anaemia in patients with lower-risk myelodysplastic syndromes: A phase 2, dose-ranging trial. The Lancet Haematology. 2018;**5**(2):e63-e72. DOI: 10.1016/S2352-3026(18)30002-4

[138] Azra R, Al-Kali A, Tibes R, et al. Rigosertib oral in transfusion dependent

lower risk myelodysplastic syndromes (LR-MDS): Optimization of dose and rate of transfusion Independence (TI) or transfusion reduction (TR) in a single-arm phase 2 study. In the 59th American Society of Hematology annual meeting and exposition, 9-12 December 2017, Atlanta, GA. Blood. 2017;**130**:1689

[139] Besarab A, Provenzano R, Hertel J, et al. Randomized placebo-controlled dose-ranging and pharmacodynamics study of roxadustat (FG-4592) to treat anemia in nondialysis-dependent chronic kidney disease (NDD-CKD) patients. Nephrology, Dialysis, Transplantation. 2015;**30**(10):1665-1673. DOI: 10.1093/ndt/gfv302

[140] Sierra J, Perez WS, Rozman C, et al. Bone marrow transplantation from HLA-identical siblings as treatment for myelodysplasia. Blood. 2002;**100**(6):1997-2004

[141] Alyea EP, Kim HT, Ho V, et al. Comparative outcome of nonmyeloablative and myeloablative allogeneic hematopoietic cell transplantation for patients older than 50 years of age. Blood. 2005;**105**:1810-1814. DOI: 10.1182/blood-2004-05-1947

[142] Saber W, Le Rademacher J, Sekeres M, et al. Multicenter biologic assignment trial comparing reduced-intensity allogeneic hematopoietic cell transplant to hypomethylating therapy or best supportive care in patients aged 50 to 75 with intermediate-2 and high-risk myelodysplastic syndrome: Blood and marrow transplant clinical trials network #1102 study rationale, design, and methods. Biology of Blood and Marrow Transplantation. 2014;**20**(10):1566-1572. DOI: 10.1016/j.bbmt.2014.06.010

[143] Della Porta MG, Alessandrino EP, Bacigalupo A, et al. Predictive factors for the outcome of allogeneic transplantation in patients with MDS stratified according to the revised IPSS-R. Blood. 2014;**123**(15):2333-2342. DOI: 10.1182/blood-2013-12-542720

[144] Festuccia M, Deeg HJ, Gooley TA, et al. Minimal identifiable disease and the role of conditioning intensity in hematopoietic cell transplantation for MDS and AML evolving from MDS. Biology of Blood and Marrow Transplantation. 2016;**22**(7):1227-1233. DOI: 10.1016/j.bbmt.2016.03.029

[145] Bejar R, Stevenson KE, Caughey B, et al. Somatic mutations predict poor outcome in patients with myelodysplastic syndrome after hematopoietic stem-cell transplantation. Journal of Clinical Oncology. 2014;**32**(25):2691-2698. DOI: 10.1200/JCO.2013.52.3381

[146] Bejar R, Stevenson K, Abdel-Wahab O, et al. Clinical effect of point mutations in myelodysplastic syndromes. The New England Journal of Medicine. 2011;**364**(26):2496-2506. DOI: 10.1056/NEJMoa1013343

Chapter 6

Noncoding RNAs in Myelodysplastic Syndromes

Andrea Hruštincová, Katarina Szikszai, Zdeněk Krejčík, Nikoleta Loudová and Michaela Dostálová Merkerová

Abstract

The discovery of short regulatory RNAs has recently directed the attention of scientists to parts of the genome that previously had been regarded as "junk" DNA because they did not encode protein products. The revelation that even protein-noncoding sequences had biological functions began the era of discovering the world of noncoding RNAs (ncRNAs). Of these ncRNAs, microRNAs (miRNAs) and long noncoding RNAs (lncRNAs) are the most numerous and best-known ncRNA groups. miRNAs and lncRNAs are important regulators of hematopoiesis, and their abnormal function has serious implications for phenotypes. Deregulation of these ncRNAs is found in hematopoietic disorders, and they also contribute to the development and progression of myelodysplastic syndromes (MDS). Properties of ncRNAs such as stability and tissue specificity make these molecules highly promising diagnostic and prognostic markers as well as interesting therapeutic targets. This chapter summarizes our knowledge on the contribution of ncRNAs to the pathogenesis of MDS and discusses their potential applicability in disease diagnostics and prognosis.

Keywords: myelodysplastic syndromes, noncoding RNAs, microRNAs, long noncoding RNAs, pathogenesis

1. Introduction

Myelodysplastic syndromes (MDS) are a heterogeneous group of clonal hematopoietic stem cell (HSC) disorders, characterized by dysplastic and ineffective blood cell production, with a tendency for transformation to acute myeloid leukemia (AML). The diagnosis is generally suspected based on the presence of an abnormal complete blood count and is confirmed by performing bone marrow (BM) aspiration and biopsy, demonstrating morphological evidence of dysplasia. A number of additional tests, including cytogenetics, flow cytometry, and molecular genetics, are needed to complete the laboratory evaluation of patients with MDS [1].

Because of the large heterogeneity of MDS, the development of additional molecular tools able to refine the prognostic scoring system, to predict outcome, and to monitor the response to treatment is required. Recently, application of new high-throughput methods such as next-generation sequencing (NGS) has identified recurrent somatic mutations in MDS cells. In particular, point mutations in the TP53, EZH2, ETV6, RUNX1, and ASXL1 genes have been shown to be associated with specific clinical features and poor overall survival, independent of established risk factors [2]. Even though approximately 78% of MDS patients carry at least one oncogenic mutation [3], there is a long list of mutations in more than 50 genes with often unclear etiology, complicating the use of somatic mutations as simple and universal markers of MDS prognosis.

Concerning MDS pathogenesis, substantial progress has been made in recent years. A vast literature has become available regarding the spectrum of cytogenetic abnormalities, gene mutations, epigenetic modifications, gene expression patterns, and deregulated signaling pathways (e.g., apoptosis, proliferation, immune response, chromatin remodeling, RNA-splicing machinery, oxidative damage/DNA repair, microenvironment interactions, and others) associated with the disease. In this review, we discuss the contributions of noncoding RNAs (ncRNAs) to the pathogenesis of MDS as well as their potential applications as novel molecular markers for clinical purposes.

2. Noncoding RNAs

At the end of the last millennium, the importance of noncoding RNAs was completely unknown. Up to that point, the scientific community focused on genes that coded for proteins. The classic dogma of molecular biology postulated that DNA was transcribed into RNA, which was then translated into protein, ignoring all non-protein-coding sequences. Only in 1993 did the importance of miRNAs begin to be revealed. The discovery of the first miRNA, lin-4, from *Caenorhabditis elegans* [4, 5] initiated a new scientific era that definitively overcame the absolute sanctity of the central dogma. Interest in this field was further stimulated by the finding that almost all of the mammalian genome was transcribed at some level [6], raising speculation that much of this pervasive transcription was likely functional. This idea was epitomized by the ENCODE (Encyclopedia of DNA Elements, www.encodeproject.org) consortium that claimed to have assigned "biochemical functions for 80% of the genome" [7, 8]. From the beginning of this era, researchers identified thousands of previously unknown types of noncoding RNAs and indeed started to reveal their multiple functions affecting various features of cells.

2.1 Types of noncoding RNAs

Functional ncRNAs can be divided into two main types: infrastructural and regulatory ncRNAs. Infrastructural ncRNAs appear to have housekeeping roles in translation and splicing; they include species such as ribosomal RNAs (rRNAs), transfer RNAs (tRNAs), and small nuclear RNAs (snRNAs) that are involved in splicing events. Regulatory ncRNAs, including long noncoding RNAs (lncRNAs), microRNAs (miRNAs), and piwi-interacting RNAs (piRNAs) are involved in the modification and interactions with other RNAs. However, ncRNAs can also be categorized on the basis of length (small, 18–31 nt; medium, 31–200 nt; and long, >200 nt), structure (circular RNAs (circRNAs)), or subcellular localization (small nuclear RNAs (snRNAs) and small nucleolar RNAs (snoRNAs)). Other infrequent ncRNA types such as trans-spliced transcripts and macroRNAs that comprise enormous genomic distances, or multigene transcripts containing several genes or even the whole chromosome, further complicate efforts at systematic classification [9]. Moreover, clear categorization of ncRNA species is difficult, as many ncRNA transcripts often share properties of several categories. The major classes of ncRNAs are summarized in **Table 1**.

ncRNA class	Description	Description	Length
rRNA	Ribosomal RNA	RNA that is directly incorporated into the ribosome	Large subunit (5S–121 nt, 5.8S–156 nt, 28S–5070 nt) Small subunit (18S–1869 nt)
tRNA	Transfer RNA	Transfer amino acids to the ribosome for protein construction	76–90 nt
snRNA	Small nuclear RNA	Small RNA located in the nucleus, involved in spliceosomes (e.g., U1, U2, U5, U4, and U6), RNA modification, and other functions. Also commonly referred to as U-RNAs	~150 nt
snoRNA	Small nucleolar RNA	RNA located in the nucleolus, mostly involved in modification of other RNAs, such as rRNA (C/D-box and H/ACA box snoRNAs) or spliceosomal RNA (scaRNA)	~60–250 nt
miRNA	microRNA	A short single-stranded RNA that usually suppresses the translation of target mRNA by binding to 3′ UTR through RNA interference pathways	21–25 nt
siRNA	Small interfering RNA	Double-stranded RNA that guides sequence-specific degradation of target mRNA through RNA interference pathway	10–25 bp
piRNA	Piwi-interacting RNA	A large class of small ncRNAs involved in retrotransposon silencing through interactions with piwi proteins	26–31 nt
Y-RNA	Y RNA	Components of the Ro ribonucleoprotein complex, repressing its activity. It is also required for DNA replication	69–112 nt
circRNA	Circular RNA	RNA derived from precursor mRNAs forming covalently closed continuous loop. It is more resistant to exonuclease-mediated degradation	1–5 exons
lncRNA	Long noncoding RNA	A non–protein-coding transcript with >200 nt	>200 nt

Table 1.
The major categories of ncRNAs.

Of the various classes of ncRNAs, miRNAs and lncRNAs are the most numerous and are probably the best-known ncRNA groups (numbers of publications concerning miRNAs and lncRNAs are shown in **Figure 1**). Having different regulatory functions, these types of ncRNAs are important players in the majority of cellular processes, including hematopoiesis, and their abnormal function has serious implications for phenotypes. Deregulation of miRNAs and lncRNAs is frequently found in hematopoietic disorders, contributing substantially to the disease development and progression. Therefore, the following sections of this review will primarily focus on these two categories of ncRNAs and their functions in MDS.

3. MicroRNAs

miRNAs are short single-stranded noncoding RNA molecules of approximately 21–25 nt in length. Their sequences are highly conserved in both plants and animals and are thought to be an evolutionarily ancient component of gene regulation. miRNAs posttranscriptionally regulate gene expression through the RNA

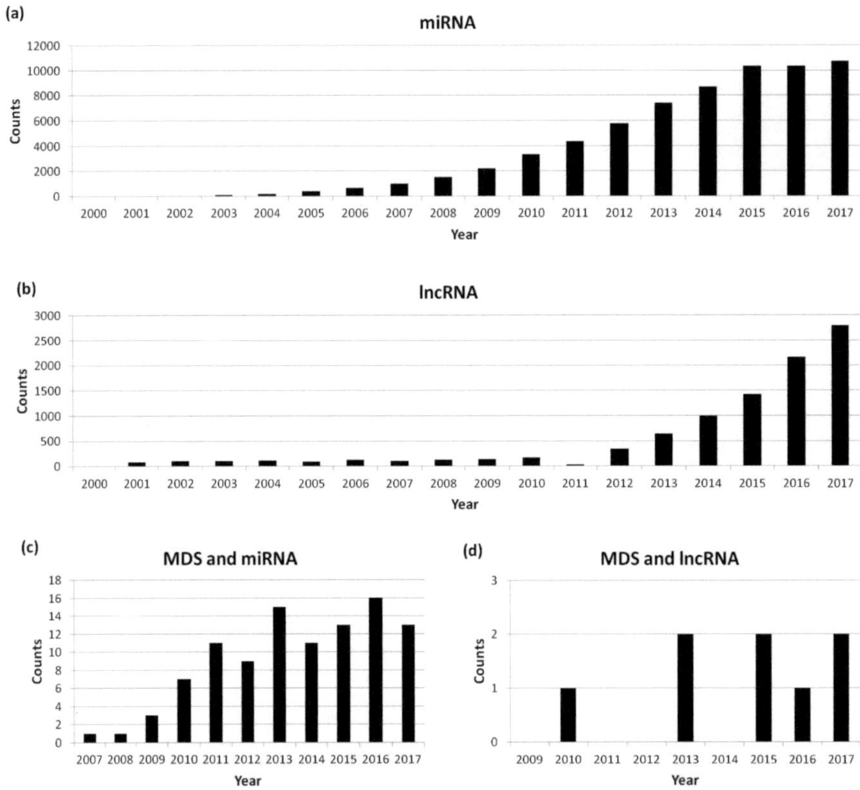

Figure 1.
Numbers of publications found on Pubmed using search terms: (a) miRNA (b) lncRNA, (c) MDS and miRNA, and (d) MDS and lncRNA (since the year 2000).

interference pathway. During the last decade, it has repeatedly been proven that miRNAs play crucial roles in a wide variety of biological processes such as development, differentiation, proliferation, and apoptosis. Because miRNAs influence the expression of genes involved in fundamental signaling pathways, their deregulation often triggers various pathological processes, including cardiovascular diseases, neurological diseases, and cancer.

The first miRNA, lin-4 from *Caenorhabditis elegans*, was discovered in the early 1990s [4, 5]. However, miRNAs were not recognized as a distinct class of biological regulators until the early 2000s. To date, thousands of miRNAs have been identified in humans and other species, and miRNA online sequence repositories, such as the miRBase database (www.mirbase.org), are available. According to the current version of the miRBase database (release 22), there are 1982 precursor miRNAs and 2693 mature miRNAs known in humans.

The biogenesis of miRNAs is a multistep process. miRNA genes are transcribed from genomic DNA by RNA polymerase II, resulting in primary miRNA (pri-miRNA) transcripts that usually encode sequences for several miRNAs. In the nucleus, these pri-miRNAs are cleaved by endonuclease Drosha, releasing approximately 70 nucleotide-long hairpin precursor miRNAs (pre-miRNAs). Pre-miRNAs are transported into the cytoplasm, where they are cleaved by Dicer into dsRNA duplexes containing both mature miRNA strand (miRNA) and its complementary strand (miRNA*). In general, the mature miRNA strands are preferentially loaded into the miRNA-induced silencing complex (miRISC), whereas the complementary strands are excluded and degraded. Once processed from the hairpin and loaded into the silencing complex, the miRNA pairs with messenger RNA (mRNA) to direct posttranscriptional repression. At sites with extensive pairing complementarity, the miRNA directs argonaute-catalyzed mRNA cleavage. More commonly, however, the miRNAs direct translational repression, mRNA destabilization, or a combination of the two [10].

It has been shown that an individual miRNA is able to control the expression of more than one target mRNA and that each mRNA may be regulated by several miRNAs. Generally, it is believed that miRNAs regulate more than 30% of protein-coding genes in the human genome [11]. The ability of miRNAs to interact with thousands of mRNAs has raised intensive interest in their role in physiological and pathological conditions. Like mRNAs, the majority of miRNAs are expressed in tissue-specific manners. For example, miR-122 is preferentially expressed in liver [12], miR-124 in neurological tissues [13], miR-133 in muscles [14], and miR-208a in heart [15]. Moreover, it has been demonstrated that changes in the spectrum of tissue miRNAs correlate with various pathophysiological conditions [16].

3.1 Extracellular miRNAs

In recent years, cell-free circulating miRNAs have been found in various body fluids such as blood, cerebrospinal fluid, saliva, and urine [17]. The first extracellular small RNAs were observed in blood in 2004 [18]. Unlike the comprehensively described function of cellular miRNAs, the function of miRNAs present in the extracellular environment remains somewhat speculative. However, a growing body of evidence has suggested that these molecules are not mere leftovers of cellular degradation without any specific functions, but that active exchange of miRNAs between cells can play an important role in long-distance cell-to-cell communication.

In 2008, Mitchell et al. [19] reported that extracellular miRNAs were stable in human plasma/serum. This high stability of circulating miRNAs despite high levels of RNase activity in blood indicates that circulating miRNAs must somehow be protected from degradation. To date, a number of miRNA carriers have been described: membrane-derived vesicles (shedding vesicles, exosomes), lipoproteins, and ribonucleoprotein complexes (with argonaute-2 (AGO2) or nucleophosmin 1 (NPM1) proteins) have been found to transport extracellular miRNAs. It has been reported that the sorting of miRNAs into various types of vesicles can be selective. Diehl et al. [20] compared the content of miRNAs in microvesicles and their maternal cells. These authors demonstrated a significantly varied spectrum of miRNAs in both samples, suggesting a selective packaging of miRNAs into microvesicles.

3.2 miRNAs in normal hematopoiesis

The differentiation and homeostasis of the hematopoietic system requires complex and interconnected molecular networks that need careful regulation. During the last decade, the role of miRNAs in the hematopoietic system has been extensively studied, and many miRNAs serving as critical regulators of both normal immune functions and diseases have been discovered (**Figure 2**).

The first study of a role of miRNAs in the differentiation of the immune system showed that forced expression of miR-181 in hematopoietic stem cells (HSCs) markedly increased the number of B lymphocytes, with a concomitant reduction of T lymphocytes [21]. Since then, other miRNAs specific for the maintenance of the "stemness" of HSCs and for the development of individual blood cell lines have been determined. For example, miR-125a was found to be sufficient as a single miRNA to

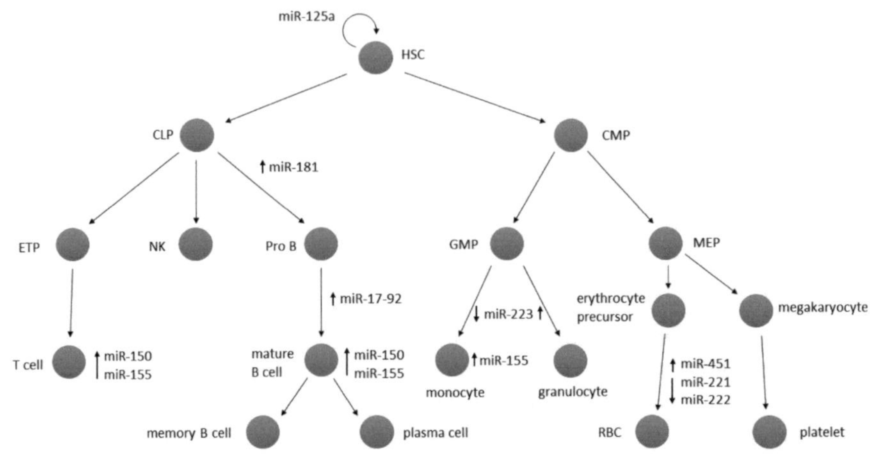

Figure 2.
Schema of lineage differentiation in hematopoiesis and miRNAs involved in the process. CLP—common lymphoid progenitor, CMP—common myeloid progenitor, ETP—early thymic progenitor, GMP—granulocyte macrophage progenitor, HSC—hematopoietic stem cell, MEP—megakaryocyte erythroid progenitor, NK—natural killer cell, RBC—red blood cell.

modulate HSC self-renewal and numbers and to protect lineage-negative progenitor cells from apoptosis [22]. A key miRNA that regulates granulocytic differentiation and function is miR-223. This miRNA shows a highly lineage-specific pattern of expression with low levels in HSCs and common myeloid progenitors. The expression of this miRNA is steadily upregulated during differentiation to granulocytes and is repressed during differentiation to the alternative monocytic fate [23]. miR-451 is expressed predominantly in erythroid cells, and its expression is significantly increased during maturation of erythrocytes. In contrast, miR-221 and miR-222 are downregulated during erythroid differentiation. This downregulation enables the expression of their target gene KIT (KIT proto-oncogene receptor tyrosine kinase, CD117), whose activation triggers erythroblast expansion [24]. Another miRNA, miR-150, is highly expressed in mature lymphocytes, whereas it is not active in HSCs. The target gene of miR-150 is transcription factor MYB (myeloblastosis) that regulates lymphocyte development [25]. miR-155, with its high levels in activated B cells, T cells, and monocytes, also participates in lymphoid differentiation. The development of B cells is positively regulated by miRNAs encoded by cluster miR-17-92. This cluster of miRNAs inhibits the expression of the apoptotic gene BIM (proapoptotic BH3-only Bcl-2 family member) and thus plays a key role in pro-B cells to pre-B cells transition [26]. In our laboratory, we analyzed miRNA expression in individual cell types from the peripheral blood of healthy individuals and determined a panel of 13 miRNAs whose expression profile enables differentiation of individual blood cell lines and determination of the cellular origin of in vitro cultured lines [27].

3.3 miRNAs in malignant hematopoiesis

In oncogenesis, miRNAs act both as oncogenes and as tumor suppressors. Mechanisms of deregulation are similar to those of protein-coding genes (chromosome aberrations, mutations, and epigenetic modifications). In 2002, the loss of two miRNAs (miR-15a and miR-16-1) due to a deletion in the 13q14 region in patients with chronic lymphocytic leukemia was described for the first time as directly associated with malignant disease [28]. In subsequent years, several miRNAs with key roles in the pathogenesis and prognosis of hematological malignancies were detected.

Several publications involved investigations of the role of miRNAs in AML. miRNA expression profiling revealed marked differences in miRNA expression between common cytogenetic subtypes of AML. Jongen-Lavrencic et al. [29] identified upregulation of several miRNAs (miR-382, miR-134, miR-376a, miR-127, miR-299-5p, and miR-323) in AML patients with t(15;17) and significant downregulation of miRNAs from let-7 family in AML with t(8;21) as well as in AML with inv(16). Moreover, miRNA signatures have been reported to be associated with recurrent molecular abnormalities in cytogenetically normal AML [30]. For example, upregulation of miR-10, let-7, and miR-29 family members and downregulation of miR-204 and miR-128a were found in AML with *NPM1* mutations [31] and high expression of miR-181a and miR-181b was associated with *CEBPA* (CCAAT/enhancer binding protein alpha) mutations [32].

3.4 miRNA deregulation in MDS

Several preliminary reports focused on identification of miRNA expression profiles that were either common in MDS or specific for individual MDS subcategories. For example, Pons et al. [33] measured levels of expression of 25 mature miRNAs in mononuclear cells (MNCs) of MDS patients. The authors reported overexpression of miRNA cluster miR-17-92 in MDS and differential expression of miR-15a and miR-16 between low- and high-risk subgroups of patients. Hussein et al. [34] showed that the miRNA profiles in BM cells discriminated MDS with chromosomal alterations from patients with normal karyotypes. Sokol et al. [35] examined miRNA signature in BM MNCs and found deregulation of several miRNAs (increase of miR-222 and miR-10a; decrease of miR-146a, miR-150, and let-7e) in MDS. In our study, we analyzed miRNA expression on a genome-wide level in $CD34^+$ BM cells. We observed significant differences in miRNA expression between early and advanced MDS; an apparent changeover was found between MDS with excess blast 1 (MDS-EB1) and MDS-EB2 subtypes. In particular, we identified strong upregulation of proapoptotic miR-34a in early subtypes of MDS [36].

Although many studies were conducted regarding miRNA profiling in MDS, there have been very few overlaps among them. This inconsistency may mirror the heterogeneity of the disease but also may possibly be explained by variations between the protocols and platforms used for miRNA detection.

There are several lines of evidence that many miRNAs are deregulated in MDS; however, the functions of miRNAs in MDS pathogenesis remain rather unknown. Identification of target genes of miRNAs in MDS and their functional proofs in both in vitro cell cultures and in vivo animal models are necessary to realizing this goal.

3.4.1 miRNAs in MDS with del(5q)

One of the best-characterized MDS subtypes is MDS with isolated del(5q), formerly referred to as 5q− syndrome. Haploinsufficiency of specific genes within common deleted region (CDR) localized in 5q31.3-5q33 locus is essential for the specific phenotype of MDS with del(5q). In addition to protein-coding genes, 13 genes encoding miRNAs are located in CDR. Most importantly, Starczynowski et al. [37] correlated del(5q) haploinsufficiency with loss of two miRNAs that are abundant in hematopoietic stem/progenitor cells (HSPCs), miR-145 and miR-146a. Knockdown of miR-145 and miR-146a together in mouse HSPCs resulted in thrombocytosis, mild neutropenia, and megakaryocytic dysplasia [37].

Kumar et al. [38] showed that miR-145 loss in MDS with del(5q) affects megakaryocyte and erythroid differentiation. These authors found that miR-145 functions through the repression of FLI1 (Friend Leukemia Integration 1 Transcription

Factor), a megakaryocyte and erythroid regulatory transcription factor. Inhibition of miR-145 increases the production of megakaryocytic cells relative to that of erythroid cells. Moreover, the authors proved that combined loss of miR-145 and RPS14 (a ribosomal gene that is required for the maturation of 40S ribosomal subunits and that maps to the CDR) cooperates to alter erythroid-megakaryocytic differentiation in a manner similar to that of the 5q- syndrome [38].

In our studies, we detected high expression of miR-34a in MDS del(5q) patients [36, 39]. The expression of miR-34a is induced by p53, activating apoptosis through inhibition of BCL2 gene (B-Cell CLL/Lymphoma 2, Apoptosis Regulator). This result is consistent with the increased apoptosis of progenitor cells seen in MDS del(5q).

3.4.2 miRNAs related to prognosis of MDS

Several publications have focused on miRNA expression in MDS with regard to prognostic potential. The earliest study in this area associated miRNA profiles with the International Prognostic Scoring System (IPSS) score [35]. A unique signature consisting of 10 miRNAs was closely associated with IPSS risk category permitting discrimination between lower- and higher-risk disease. Selective overexpression of miR-181 family members was detected in higher risk MDS, indicating pathogenetic overlap with AML. Survival analysis revealed shorter survival in patients with high expression of miR-181 family than in patients with low miR-181 expression [35].

Another miRNA that has been identified as having prognostic value in MDS is miR-22 [40]. This miRNA was upregulated in MDS and its level correlated with poor survival. Transgenic mice expressing miR-22 in the hematopoietic cells displayed reduced levels of global 5-hydroxymethylcytosine and increased HSC self-renewal accompanied by defective differentiation. Over time, these mice developed MDS. Interestingly, TET2 gene (Ten-Eleven Translocation 2, Tet Methylcytosine Dioxygenase 2) was identified as a key target of miR-22 in this context [40]. TET2 is a major regulator of DNA demethylation by conversion of methylated cytosine into 5-hydroxymethylcytosine.

3.4.3 miRNAs in the treatment of MDS

Expression profiles of miRNAs also appear to be applicable predictors of treatment responses. Lenalidomide is an immunomodulatory and antiangiogenic agent used for the treatment of MDS with del(5q). In recent years, several studies have analyzed miRNA expression levels before and after lenalidomide treatment in these patients [41–44]. Oliva et al. [41] investigated expression of selected genes/miRNAs at baseline and after 3 and 6 months of lenalidomide treatment. These authors showed that the expression levels of miR-145, miR-146, and miR-155 gradually increased during the course of the treatment. The significant role of miR-143 and miR-145 in response to lenalidomide was confirmed by Venner et al. [42], who showed that lenalidomide selectively abrogated progenitor activity in cells depleted of miR-143 and miR-145, supporting their key role in the sensitivity to lenalidomide in MDS with del(5q). In our studies, the most significant changes in expression levels (decreases) after lenalidomide treatment showed miR-34a and several miRNAs clustered within the 14q32 locus [43, 44]. However, a question remains as to whether the changes in expression levels were due to direct response to lenalidomide or whether they were caused by a reduction of the pathological clone.

Therapy with hypomethylating agents (HMAs) such as azacitidine and decitabine is currently considered to be the standard therapy for higher-risk MDS and AML with myelodysplasia-related changes. Several studies investigated miRNA expression with respect to HMA treatment in AML [45–47]. Blum et al. [45] proposed miR-29b as a predictive factor for the stratification of older AML patients treated with decitabine; however, this was not confirmed by other studies [46]. Butrym et al. [47] showed that low expression of miR-181 at diagnosis was a predictor of complete remission and prolonged survival in a subset of older AML patients treated with azacitidine.

In relation to HMA therapy in MDS, it was found that the level of extracellular miR-21 was associated with overall response rate and progression-free survival [48]. Furthermore, reduced expression of miR-124 (caused by abnormal methylation) was found in MDS/AML patients responding to decitabine. These patients exhibited significantly lower expression levels of the CDK6 gene (cyclin-dependent kinase 6) that is the target of miR-124 [49]. Moreover, hypermethylation of miR-124-3p gene appeared to be a good prognostic marker of overall survival [50]. In our report, we found that the overall response rate to azacitidine treatment was significantly higher in MDS/AML patients with upregulated miR-17-3p and downregulated miR-100-5p and miR-133b and that the high level of miR-100-5p was associated with shorter overall survival [51].

3.4.4 Extracellular miRNAs in MDS

To date, only a few studies have investigated circulating miRNAs in MDS [48, 52–54]. Two papers [48, 52] focused on specific circulating miRNAs (miR-21, let-7a, and miR-16) that were preselected based on information regarding their deregulation in blood cells and their importance in similar diseases. Researchers monitored the plasma/serum levels of these miRNAs and showed that their levels could serve as prognostic markers for MDS. Kim et al. [48] showed that serum level of miR-21 was significantly associated with overall response rate and progression-free survival in MDS patients treated with HMAs. The publication that studied let-7a and miR-16 demonstrated that high plasma levels of these miRNAs can serve as semi-invasive markers of poor outcome for MDS patients [52].

Zuo et al. [53] measured expression of 800 human miRNAs in MDS plasma. These authors identified a 7-miRNA signature (let-7a, miR-144, miR-16, miR-25, miR-451, miR-651, and miR-655) as an independent predictor of survival in MDS patients with normal karyotypes.

In our study, we investigated the spectrum (2006 human miRNAs) of circulating miRNAs in the plasma of MDS patients [54]. With regard to prognosis, the levels of miR-27a-3p, miR-150-5p, miR-199a-5p, miR-223-3p, and miR-451a were lower in higher risk MDS. Moreover, miR-451a was an independent predictor of progression-free survival, and there was a significant association of miR-223-3p with overall survival [54].

These pioneer studies suggested that plasma levels of specific miRNAs were associated with MDS patient outcome and may add information beyond the currently used scoring systems. Despite these early promising results, there remain insufficient data regarding the full spectrum of extracellular RNAs in MDS. To date, the possible presence of various forms of small noncoding RNAs (apart from mature miRNAs), pathways for their protection, and identification of their cells of origin have not been explored in MDS. These missing information would expand the knowledge regarding extracellular RNAs in this disease, and beyond that, it would definitely contribute to better interpretation of alterations of individual miRNAs with the potential to become specific prognostic markers in MDS.

4. Long noncoding RNAs

lncRNAs form perhaps the most numerous group of ncRNAs. These RNAs are defined as protein-noncoding transcripts longer than 200 nucleotides. This length was proposed to distinguish lncRNAs from small noncoding RNAs. In contrast with protein-coding RNAs, lncRNAs contain only short open reading frames or completely lack them. This group of ncRNAs is characterized by high levels of structural and functional diversity, low levels of GC nucleotides, and lower expression levels, in contrast with protein-coding transcripts. lncRNAs are transcribed by RNA polymerase II or III and subsequently can be spliced and polyadenylated at the 3′ end or may contain a 5′ cap, depending on their biogenesis. Their expression is developmental and tissue-specific.

Some lncRNAs regulate (negatively or positively) the expression of genes in *trans* or *cis* by affecting RNA polymerase II recruitment or by inducing chromatin remodeling. In addition, antisense transcripts can pair with their specific sense RNA, facilitating alternative splicing. When lncRNAs interact with proteins, they can influence protein activity or localization or even help to form cellular substructures or ribonucleoprotein complexes. lncRNAs can be processed to yield small, single- or double-stranded RNAs that can act as endogenous small interfering RNAs (siRNAs) or miRNAs. Moreover, they can also act as "miRNA sponges" that affect the competitive endogenous RNA (ceRNA) network. However, additional functions and detailed signaling pathways of lncRNAs remain to be clarified [55].

According to their position relative to protein-coding mRNAs, lncRNAs are further subcategorized into several groups. Long intergenic noncoding RNAs (lincRNAs) are lncRNAs that are located between annotated protein-coding genes and that are at least 1 kb away from the nearest protein-coding genes. Intronic lncRNAs are coded within introns of protein-coding genes. Sense and antisense lncRNAs are transcribed from the sense or antisense strands of protein-coding genes and often contain exons of this gene with mutual overlap. Bidirectional lncRNAs are oriented head-to-head with protein-coding genes within 1 kb. Bidirectional lncRNA transcripts often exhibit similar expression patterns to those of their protein-coding counterpart, suggesting that they may be subject to shared regulatory pressures. Another group of lncRNA is TERRA (Telomeric Repeat-Containing RNA), transcribed from constitutive heterochromatin-rich regions, or T-UCR (Transcribed Ultraconserved Regions), transcribed from highly conserved regions of the genome.

Although more than 100,000 lncRNAs have been identified to date, only a small number of them have been characterized in detail. To integrate the data describing various lncRNAs, their expression profiles, molecular features, and functions in a variety of cell systems, several databases containing a comprehensive list of lncRNAs have been developed and are continually being updated. Among the most comprehensive databases are LNCipedia (compendium of human lncRNAs, lncipedia.org) [56], lncRNAdb (reference database for functional lncRNAs, lncRNAdb.org) [57], and NRED (database of lncRNA expression, nred.matticklab.com) [58].

4.1 lncRNAs in normal hematopoiesis

Recently, lncRNAs have emerged as important regulators of cell fate. These RNAs play a variety of roles in controlling various steps in hematopoietic differentiation, including maintenance of HSCs and differentiation of myeloid, erythroid, and lymphoid lineages. To date, there have been several descriptions of lncRNAs crucial for correct function of the hematopoietic system (**Table 2**). The first hematopoiesis-associated lncRNA, EGOT (Eosinophil Granule Ontogeny Transcript), was described in 2007. EGOT, a conserved transcript localized antisense to ITPR1 (Inositol 1,4,5-Trisphosphate Receptor Type 1) that modulates the development of eosinophils, is normally expressed in human CD34$^+$ HSCs, and its expression level increases during eosinophil development, helping to regulate production of eosinophil granule proteins [59].

The relatively well-known lncRNA, H19, maintains quiescence of adult HSCs. The H19 transcript was in fact the first lncRNA to be identified, enriched in the embryonic fetal liver but downregulated after birth [60]. H19 is active in long-term HSCs and becomes gradually downregulated in short-term HSCs and multipotent progenitors. Deletion of H19 from the maternal allele resulted in increased HSC activation and proliferation as well as impaired repopulating ability. This effect is mediated by derepression of maternal IGF2 (Insulin-Like Growth Factor 2) expression and by increased IGF1R (IGF1 Receptor) translation, resulting in increased signaling through the IGF1R [61].

Zhang et al. [62] identified HOTAIRM1 (Homeobox Antisense Intergenic RNA Myeloid 1), which is encoded within the human HOXA (Homeobox A) gene cluster and plays a role in the differentiation of myeloid cells. The expression of this transcript is upregulated during granulocyte differentiation. Knockdown of HOTAIRM1 reduced transcription of HOXA1 and HOXA4 in an acute promyelocytic leukemia cell line, resulting in a decreased expression of genes associated with granulocyte activation, defense response, and maturation [62].

LncRNA	Localization	Function	Reference
EGOT (Eosinophil Granule Ontogeny Transcript)	3p26.1, antisense to ITPR1 gene	Modulates development of eosinophils	[59]
H19	11p15.5, antisense to IGF2	Maintains quiescence of adult HSCs	[60]
HOTAIRM (Hox Antisense Intergenic RNA Myeloid 1)	7p15.2, encoded within the HOXA gene cluster	Induces differentiation of myeloid cells	[62]
lincRNA-EPS	Mouse 4qC7	Promotes red blood cell maturation	[63]
T-ALL-R-LncR1	6q24.3	Induces apoptosis in T-ALL	[66]
LUNAR1 (Leukemia-Induced Noncoding Activator RNA)	15q26.3	Positive regulator of cell division	[67]
HOTAIR (Hox Transcript Antisense RNA)	12q13.13, encoded within the HOXC gene cluster	Oncogene, promotes chromatin relocalization	[68]
MALAT-1 (Metastasis Associated Lung Adenocarcinoma Transcript)	11q13.1	Regulates transcription and cell cycle	[69]
MEG3 (Maternally Expressed Gene 3)	14q32.2	Tumor suppressor	[70]
XIST (X-Inactive Specific Transcript)	Xq13.2	Regulates X chromosome inactivation during embryogenesis	[73]

Table 2.
Examples of lncRNAs involved in normal and malignant hematopoiesis.

Hu et al. [63] studied the lncRNA transcriptome of the erythroid lineage and uncovered numerous erythroid-specific lncRNAs that become induced during terminal differentiation of mouse fetal liver red blood cells in vivo. These authors showed that lincRNA-EPS (erythroid prosurvival) acts to promote red blood cell maturation by downregulating proapoptotic pathways. Knockdown of lincRNA-EPS severely compromised terminal differentiation of erythroid progenitors and resulted in elevated apoptosis. Conversely, its ectopic expression protected erythroid progenitors from apoptosis triggered by erythropoietin starvation. Functional studies indicated that lincRNA-EPS acts by repressing a number of proapoptotic proteins, most prominently the caspase-activating adaptor protein Pycard [63].

Recent studies have also provided evidence for the importance of several lncRNAs in immune cell function. For example, lncRNA NeST (Nettoie Salmonella pas Theiler's, cleanup Salmonella not Theiler's), also named Tmevpg1, modulates the ability of mice to respond to viral and bacterial infections. NeST is specifically expressed by the T_H1 subset of helper T cells. The expression of NeST regulates the degree of inflammation induced by infecting pathogens, such as Thelier's virus or Salmonella [64]. lncRNA-Cox2 (cyclooxygenase 2) acts during inflammatory signaling by modulating the expression of several immune response genes via interactions with regulatory complexes [65].

4.2 lncRNAs in malignant hematopoiesis

lncRNAs not only participate in normal hematopoiesis but also contribute to the pathogenesis of hematologic malignancies, representing a new class of potential biomarkers and therapeutic targets. These RNAs have significantly different expression levels in primary tumors and metastases, functioning both as oncogenes or as tumor suppressors. Some cancer-related lncRNAs could affect the development and progression of tumor by means of p53, polycomb repressive complex 2 (PRC2), and other signaling pathways. Others are not observed in normal tissue but are detected in cancer. For example, T-ALL-R-lncR1 appears to induce (together with protease-activated receptor 4 (PAR-4)) cellular apoptosis in T cell acute lymphoblastic leukemia cells (T-ALL) [66]. LUNAR1 (leukemia-induced noncoding activator RNA) is highly expressed in T-ALL cells, and its expression is dependent on signaling through the oncogenic NOTCH1 receptor [67]. lncRNAs HOTAIR (homeobox transcript antisense RNA) and MALAT-1 (metastasis-associated lung adenocarcinoma transcript) are associated with metastasis and recurrence [68, 69].

4.2.1 lncRNA deregulation in MDS

The first study describing lncRNA in the context of MDS was published in 2010 by Benetatos et al. [70] who studied lncRNA MEG3 (maternally expressed gene 3). Abnormal methylation of its promoter was observed in a third of MDS patients and in half of AML patients [70]. MEG3 was the first lncRNA described to have a tumor suppressor function. MEG3 is expressed in many human normal tissues, and numerous studies have demonstrated that its expression level is lost in various cancers. Low expression of MEG3 is associated with an increased risk of metastasis and poor prognosis in cancer patients [71, 72].

In 2013, Yildirim et al. [73] conditionally deleted lncRNA XIST (X-inactive specific transcript) in mice hematopoietic cells. XIST is perhaps the most well-understood lncRNA to date. This lncRNA is located on the X chromosome and is required for X chromosome inactivation during embryogenesis. Yildirim et al. [73]

demonstrated that mutant females developed a highly aggressive myeloproliferative neoplasm and MDS (mixed MPN/MDS) with 100% penetrance.

The first study examining the deregulation of lncRNAs on a genome-wide level in MDS was published in 2017 [74]. The authors combined NGS and microarray data in $CD34^+$ BM cells and identified several lncRNAs (linc-ARFIP1-4, linc-TAAR9-1, lincC2orf85, linc-RNFT2-1, and linc-RPIA) deregulated in MDS-EB2. In the same year, Yao et al. [75] profiled lncRNA expressions in 176 adult patients with primary MDS and identified four lncRNAs (TC07000551.hg.1, TC08000489.hg.1, TC02004770.hg.1, and TC03000701) with expression levels significantly associated with overall survival. Subsequently, the authors constructed a risk-scoring system with the weighted sum of these four lncRNAs. Higher lncRNA scores were associated with higher marrow blast percentages, higher-risk subtypes of MDS, complex cytogenetic changes, and mutations in RUNX1, ASXL1, TP53, SRSF2, and ZRSR2, whereas they were inversely correlated with the SF3B1 mutation. Patients with higher lncRNA scores had significantly shorter overall survival and higher 5-year leukemic transformation rate than did those with lower scores [75].

Although increasing numbers of deregulated lncRNAs are currently being described in MDS, only a few have been functionally characterized so far. Transcriptomic data may be used to construct network modules consisting of lncRNAs and protein-coding genes to enable functional analysis of lncRNAs with unknown functions. These networks are subsequently linked with annotated signaling pathways and gene ontologies. The resulting outputs provide a degree of functional annotation for differentially expressed lncRNAs in the disease and their potential roles in pathophysiology [74].

5. Other types of noncoding RNAs in MDS

Only very limited information regarding other groups of ncRNAs have been published for MDS to date. However, we can anticipate that introduction of next-generation sequencing of RNAs (so-called RNA-seq) will bring to MDS research many novel insights regarding various ncRNAs in the near future. This technology enables sensitive global detection of various RNAs across an unparalleled dynamic range. Particularly, small RNA-seq is predominantly used for detection of miRNAs. However, during library preparation, small RNAs are selected by electrophoresis with sizes typically ranging from 20 to 50 nt. This range of size selection allows for the capture of many other species of small RNAs in addition to miRNAs.

5.1 Piwi-interacting RNAs

In 2011, Beck et al. [76] conducted one of the early studies to apply small RNA-seq in MDS. These authors compared expression of small RNAs between low-grade (refractory anemia, RA) and high-grade (MDS-EB2) MDS patients and demonstrated the first evidence of piwi (P-element-Induced Wimpy Testis)-interacting RNAs (piRNAs) in MDS BM cells and their particular enrichment in low-grade MDS. PiRNAs are a relatively newly defined class of small ncRNAs with lengths from 26 to 32 nt. These RNAs lack sequence conservation and are more complex than miRNAs. PiRNAs have been linked to both epigenetic and posttranscriptional gene silencing of retrotransposons and other genetic elements in germline cells, particularly those involved in spermatogenesis.

Transcription of particular piwi proteins (*piwil1* and *piwil2*) that are required for the accumulation of piRNAs was also significantly upregulated in RA [76]. Recent studies indicated that the piwi-piRNA complex may have a role in posttranscriptional silencing of damaged DNA fragments and that interrupting piwi-piRNA formation can lead to DNA double-strand breaks [77]. In summary, the study from Beck et al. [76] suggested that the enrichment of piRNAs in low-grade MDS may potentially protect DNA from the accumulation of mutations, a mechanism not observed in high-grade MDS. Moreover, they proposed that piRNAs might be used as diagnostic markers for low-grade MDS; however, further studies of piRNA roles in MDS pathogenesis are warranted.

5.2 Transfer RNAs

The abovementioned pioneer study from Beck et al. [76] also provided an early insight into the deregulation of tRNAs in MDS. The authors showed that ratios of tRNA to rRNA were significantly higher in MDS-EB2 compared to those of RA and controls. Because tRNAs are building blocks for protein synthesis and are required during translation, this may indicate an increased regulation of translation at this disease stage. Interestingly, a significant increase of tRNAs in tumor samples was reported by Pavon-Eternod et al. [78] In addition, tRNAs have been shown to inhibit cytochrome c-activated apoptosis [79]. Taken together, Beck et al. [76] hypothesized that high tRNA content seen in EB2 may contribute to the two well-known characteristics of high-grade MDS, decreased apoptosis, and high rate of leukemic transformation.

Guo et al. [80] performed small RNA-seq in paired pre- and posttreatment samples from MDS patients receiving therapy with HMAs. In the sequencing data, the number of reads aligned to tRNA-derived small RNAs (tDRs) (78.81%) vastly outnumbered those aligning to miRNAs (4.43% of reads). The tRNA fragments that were captured by miRNA-seq might be a result of either active cleavage or artifacts of the miRNA-seq library construction. The authors identified six tDR fragments that were differentially expressed between MDS and normal samples. Three tDRs demonstrated increased expression in MDS (chrM.tRNA10.TC, chr12.tRNA8.AlaTGC, and chr16.tRNA4.ProAGG), while three were decreased (chr1.tRNA58-LeuCAA, chr19.tRNA8-SeC(e)TCA (SeC(e)TCA), and chr19.tRNA4-ThrAGT). Moreover, they identified a panel of four tRNA fragments (chr6.tRNA157.ValCAC, chr11.tRNA17.ValTAC, chrM.tRNA12.TS1, and chrX.tRNA4.ValTAC), whose combined expression in the pretreatment samples together was predictive of the likelihood of response. Deeper focus on mitochondrial tRNAs revealed that MT-TS1 (mitochondrially encoded tRNA serine 1) was the only mitochondrial tRNA to have a significant association with treatment response [80].

6. Conclusions

The discovery of ncRNAs has initiated a new era in molecular biology, completely changing our view of "junk" DNA that it is no longer considered unnecessary ballast. Mouse models have clearly demonstrated key functions of ncRNAs in regulatory networks and their ability to significantly influence biological processes. In the hematopoietic system, ncRNAs represent important regulators of HSC "stemness" and differentiation; therefore, it is not surprising that deregulation of ncRNAs also occurs in MDS.

Currently, we possess comprehensive information regarding the impact of miRNA deregulation on the pathogenesis of MDS. The efforts of current research activities aim to apply these findings to clinical practice, testing the potential diagnostic/prognostic value of selected miRNAs for MDS. However, miRNAs also represent promising therapeutic agents or targets. miRNA-based drugs are designed to reduce the expression of oncogenic miRNAs or, conversely, to increase levels of miRNAs with tumor suppressor functions. Unlike targeted inhibition or activation of a single protein-coding gene, the administration of miRNA antagonists or their mimics may potentially improve the desired effects, as these molecules can regulate several genes, often in specific signaling pathways implicated in tumorigenesis. Several pharmaceutical companies already have miRNA therapeutics in their developmental pipelines [81]. In 2012, the first cancer-targeted miRNA drug, MRX34 (a liposome-based miR-34 mimic), entered phase I clinical trials in patients with advanced hepatocellular carcinoma, and this mimic has attracted considerable attention from both academic researchers and pharmaceutical companies [82]. MRG-106, a synthetic antagonist of miRNA-155, is currently being tested by MIRagen Therapeutics in patients with cutaneous T-cell lymphoma [83]. However, testing miRNAs as potential therapeutic agents or targets in MDS therapy still requires initial exploration in in vitro models before evolving to future clinical trials.

Information regarding the contribution of other categories of ncRNAs, including lncRNAs, to the pathogenesis of MDS remains scarce. However, given the large number of ncRNAs encoded in the human genome and the complexity of their interactions, it can be expected that, in the near future, we will reveal a number of ncRNAs involved in MDS. It can also be anticipated that we will identify new predictive markers of progression and responses to therapy among these molecules.

To conclude, the diagnostic and therapeutic possibilities of ncRNAs undoubtedly have profound potential in MDS. However, although the effects of some miRNAs have already been demonstrated, it is certain that the importance of ncRNAs in MDS will be fully understood only in the future and that many years of research and clinical trials remain before the eventual application of ncRNAs in clinical practice to classify, monitor, and treat this disease.

Acknowledgements

This work was supported by the research grants no. 16-33617A and 17-31398A and the project for conceptual development of research organization no. 00023736 (all from the Ministry of Health of the Czech Republic).

Conflict of interests

The authors declare that they have no competing interests.

Author details

Andrea Hruštincová†, Katarina Szikszai†, Zdeněk Krejčík, Nikoleta Loudová and Michaela Dostálová Merkerová*
Department of Genomics, Institute of Hematology and Blood Transfusion, Prague, Czech Republic

*Address all correspondence to: michaela.merkerova@uhkt.cz

†These authors contributed equally to this work.

References

[1] Garcia-Manero G. Myelodysplastic syndromes: 2014 update on diagnosis, risk-stratification, and management. American Journal of Hematology. 2014; **89**:97-108. DOI: 10.1002/ajh.23642

[2] Bejar R, Stevenson K, Abdel-Wahab O, Galili N, Nilsson B, Garcia-Manero G, et al. Clinical effect of point mutations in myelodysplastic syndromes. The New England Journal of Medicine. 2011;**364**:2496-2506. DOI: 10.1056/NEJMoa1013343

[3] Papaemmanuil E, Gerstung M, Malcovati L, Tauro S, Gundem G, Van Loo P, et al. Clinical and biological implications of driver mutations in myelodysplastic syndromes. Blood. 2013;**122**:3616-3627. DOI: 10.1182/blood-2013-08-518886

[4] Lee RC, Feinbaum RL, Ambros V. The *C. elegans* heterochronic gene lin-4 encodes small RNAs with antisense complementarity to lin-14. Cell. 1993;**75**: 843-854

[5] Wightman B, Ha I, Ruvkun G. Posttranscriptional regulation of the heterochronic gene lin-14 by lin-4 mediates temporal pattern formation in *C. elegans*. Cell. 1993;**75**:855-862

[6] Pennisi E. Genomics. ENCODE project writes eulogy for junk DNA. Science. 2012;**337**:1159-1161. DOI: 10.1126/science.337.6099.1159

[7] ENCODE Project Consortium. An integrated encyclopedia of DNA elements in the human genome. Nature. 2012;**489**:57-74. DOI: 10.1038/nature11247

[8] Palazzo AF, Lee ES. Non-coding RNA: What is functional and what is junk? Frontiers in Genetics. 2015;**6**:2. DOI: 10.3389/fgene.2015.00002

[9] Dozmorov MG, Giles CB, Koelsch KA, Wren JD. Systematic classification of non-coding RNAs by epigenomic similarity. BMC Bioinformatics. 2013;**14** (Suppl 14):S2. DOI: 10.1186/1471-2105-14-S14-S

[10] Bartel DP. MicroRNA target recognition and regulatory functions. Cell. 2009;**136**:215-233. DOI: 10.1016/j.cell.2009.01.002

[11] Lewis BP, Burge CB, Bartel DP. Conserved seed pairing, often flanked by adenosines, indicates that thousands of human genes are microRNA targets. Cell. 2005;**120**:15-20. DOI: 10.1016/j.cell.2004.12.035

[12] Lewis AP, Jopling CL. Regulation and biological function of the liver-specific miR-122. Biochemical Society Transactions. 2010;**38**:1553-1557. DOI: 10.1042/BST0381553

[13] Sun AX, Crabtree GR, Yoo AS. MicroRNAs: Regulators of neuronal fate. Current Opinion in Cell Biology. 2013;**25**:215-221. DOI: 10.1016/j.ceb.2012.12.007

[14] Luo W, Nie Q, Zhang X. MicroRNAs involved in skeletal muscle differentiation. Journal of Genetics and Genomics. 2013;**40**:107-116. DOI: 10.1016/j.jgg.2013.02.002

[15] van Rooij E, Sutherland LB, Qi X, Richardson JA, Hill J, Olson EN. Control of stress-dependent cardiac growth and gene expression by a microRNA. Science. 2007;**316**:575-579. DOI: 10.1126/science.1139089

[16] Lu J, Getz G, Miska EA, Alvarez-Saavedra E, Lamb J, Peck D, et al. MicroRNA expression profiles classify human cancers. Nature. 2005;**435**:834-838. DOI: 10.1038/nature03702

[17] Weber JA, Baxter DH, Zhang S, Huang DY, Huang KH, Lee MJ, et al. The microRNA spectrum in 12 body fluids. Clinical Chemistry. 2010;**56**:1733-1741. DOI: 10.1373/clinchem.2010.147405

[18] El-Hefnawy T, Raja S, Kelly L, Bigbee WL, Kirkwood JM, Luketich JD, et al. Characterization of amplifiable, circulating RNA in plasma and its potential as a tool for cancer diagnostics. Clinical Chemistry. 2004;**50**:564-573. DOI: 10.1373/clinchem.2003.028506

[19] Mitchell PS, Parkin RK, Kroh EM, Fritz BR, Wyman SK, Pogosova-Agadjanyan EL, et al. Circulating microRNAs as stable blood-based markers for cancer detection. Proceedings of the National Academy of Sciences of the United States of America. 2008;**105**:10513-10518. DOI: 10.1073/pnas.0804549105

[20] Diehl P, Fricke A, Sander L, Stamm J, Bassler N, Htun N, et al. Microparticles: Major transport vehicles for distinct microRNAs in circulation. Cardiovascular Research. 2012;**93**:633-644. DOI: 10.1093/cvr/cvs007

[21] Chen CZ, Li L, Lodish HF, Bartel DP. MicroRNAs modulate hematopoietic lineage differentiation. Science. 2004;**303**:83-86. DOI: 10.1126/science.1091903

[22] Guo S, Lu J, Schlanger R, Zhang H, Wang JY, Fox MC, et al. MicroRNA miR-125a controls hematopoietic stem cell number. Proceedings of the National Academy of Sciences of the United States of America. 2010;**107**: 14229-14234. DOI: 10.1073/pnas.0913574107

[23] Johnnidis JB, Harris MH, Wheeler RT, Stehling-Sun S, Lam MH, Kirak O, et al. Regulation of progenitor cell proliferation and granulocyte function by microRNA-223. Nature. 2008;**451**: 1125-1129. DOI: 10.1038/nature06607

[24] Bruchova H, Yoon D, Agarwal AM, Mendell J, Prchal JT. Regulated expression of microRNAs in normal and polycythemia vera erythropoiesis. Experimental Hematology. 2007;**35**: 1657-1667. DOI: 10.1016/j.exphem.2007.08.021

[25] Morris VA, Zhang A, Yang T, Stirewalt DL, Ramamurthy R, Meshinchi S, et al. MicroRNA-150 expression induces myeloid differentiation of human acute leukemia cells and normal hematopoietic progenitors. PLoS One. 2013;**8**(9): e75815. DOI: 10.1371/journal.pone.0075815

[26] Vasilatou D, Papageorgiou S, Pappa V, Papageorgiou E, Dervenoulas J. The role of microRNAs in normal and malignant hematopoiesis. European Journal of Haematology. 2010;**84**:1-16. DOI: 10.1111/j.1600-0609.2009.01348.x

[27] Merkerova M, Belickova M, Bruchova H. Differential expression of microRNAs in hematopoietic cell lineages. European Journal of Haematology. 2008;**81**:304-310. DOI: 10.1111/j.1600-0609.2008.01111.x

[28] Calin GA, Dumitru CD, Shimizu M, Bichi R, Zupo S, Noch E, et al. Frequent deletions and down-regulation of micro-RNA genes miR15 and miR16 at 13q14 in chronic lymphocytic leukemia. Proceedings of the National Academy of Sciences of the United States of America. 2002;**99**:15524-15529. DOI: 10.1073/pnas.242606799

[29] Jongen-Lavrencic M, Sun SM, Dijkstra MK, Valk PJ, Löwenberg B. MicroRNA expression profiling in relation to the genetic heterogeneity of acute myeloid leukemia. Blood. 2008; **111**:5078-5085. DOI: 10.1182/blood-2008-01-133355

[30] Zhao H, Wang D, Du W, Gu D, Yang R. MicroRNA and leukemia: Tiny molecule, great function. Critical

Reviews in Oncology/Hematology. 2010;**74**:149-155. DOI: 10.1016/j.critrevonc.2009.05.001

[31] Marcucci G, Maharry K, Radmacher MD, Mrózek K, Vukosavljevic T, Paschka P, et al. Prognostic significance of, gene and microRNA expression signatures associated with, CEBPA mutations in cytogenetically normal acute myeloid leukemia with high-risk molecular features: A Cancer and Leukemia Group B Study. Journal of Clinical Oncology. 2008;**26**:5078-5087. DOI: 10.1200/JCO.2008.17.5554

[32] Garzon R, Volinia S, Liu CG, Fernandez-Cymering C, Palumbo T, Pichiorri F, et al. MicroRNA signatures associated with cytogenetics and prognosis in acute myeloid leukemia. Blood. 2008;**111**:3183-3189. DOI: 10.1182/blood-2007-07-098749

[33] Pons A, Nomdedeu B, Navarro A, Gaya A, Gel B, Diaz T, et al. Hematopoiesis-related microRNA expression in myelodysplastic syndromes. Leukemia & Lymphoma. 2009;**50**:1854-1859. DOI: 10.3109/10428190903147645

[34] Hussein K, Theophile K, Büsche G, Schlegelberger B, Göhring G, Kreipe H, et al. Aberrant microRNA expression pattern in myelodysplastic bone marrow cells. Leukemia Research. 2010;**34**:1169-1174. DOI: 10.1016/j.leukres.2010.04.012

[35] Sokol L, Caceres G, Volinia S, Alder H, Nuovo GJ, Liu CG, et al. Identification of a risk dependent microRNA expression signature in myelodysplastic syndromes. British Journal of Haematology. 2011;**153**:24-32. DOI: 10.1111/j.1365-2141.2011.08581.x

[36] Dostalova Merkerova M, Krejcik Z, Votavova H, Belickova M, Vasikova A, Cermak J. Distinctive microRNA expression profiles in $CD34^+$ bone marrow cells from patients with myelodysplastic syndrome. European Journal of Human Genetics. 2011;**19**:313-319. DOI: 10.1038/ejhg.2010.209

[37] Starczynowski DT, Kuchenbauer F, Argiropoulos B, Sung S, Morin R, Muranyi A, et al. Identification of miR-145 and miR-146a as mediators of the 5q - syndrome phenotype. Nature Medicine. 2010;**16**:49-58. DOI: 10.1038/nm.2054

[38] Kumar MS, Narla A, Nonami A, Mullally A, Dimitrova N, Ball B, et al. Coordinate loss of a microRNA and protein-coding gene cooperate in the pathogenesis of 5q− syndrome. Blood. 2011;**118**(17):4666-4673. DOI: 10.1182/blood-2010-12-324715

[39] Votavova H, Grmanova M, Dostalova Merkerova M, Belickova M, Vasikova A, Neuwirtova R, et al. Differential expression of microRNAs in $CD34^+$ cells of 5q− syndrome. Journal of Hematology & Oncology. 2011;**4**:1. DOI: 10.1186/1756-8722-4-1

[40] Song SJ, Ito K, Ala U, Kats L, Webster K, Sun SM, et al. The oncogenic microRNA miR-22 targets the TET2 tumor suppressor to promote hematopoietic stem cell self-renewal and transformation. Cell Stem Cell. 2013;**13**:87-101. DOI: 10.1016/j.stem.2013.06.003

[41] Oliva EN, Cuzzola M, Aloe Spiriti MA, Poloni A, Laganà C, Rigolino C, et al. Biological activity of lenalidomide in myelodysplastic syndromes with del5q: Results of gene expression profiling from a multicenter phase II study. Annals of Hematology. 2013;**92**:25-32. DOI: 10.1007/s00277-012-1569-0

[42] Venner CP, Woltosz JW, Nevill TJ, Deeg HJ, Caceres G, Platzbecker U, et al. Correlation of clinical response and response duration with miR-145 induction by lenalidomide in CD34(+) cells from patients with del(5q) myelodysplastic syndrome.

Haematologica. 2013;**98**:409-413. DOI: 10.3324/haematol.2012.066068

[43] Merkerova MD, Krejcik Z, Belickova M, Hrustincova A, Klema J, Stara E, et al. Genome-wide miRNA profiling in myelodysplastic syndrome with del(5q) treated with lenalidomide. European Journal of Haematology. 2015; **95**:35-43. DOI: 10.1111/ejh.12458

[44] Krejčík Z, Beličková M, Hruštincová A, Kléma J, Zemanová Z, Michalová K, et al. Aberrant expression of the microRNA cluster in 14q32 is associated with del(5q) myelodysplastic syndrome and lenalidomide treatment. Cancer Genetics. 2015;**208**:156-161. DOI: 10.1016/j.cancergen.2015.03.003

[45] Blum W, Garzon R, Klisovic RB, Schwind S, Walker A, Geyer S, et al. Clinical response and miR-29b predictive significance in older AML patients treated with a 10-day schedule of decitabine. Proceedings of the National Academy of Sciences of the United States of America. 2010;**107**: 7473-7478. DOI: 10.1073/pnas.1002650107

[46] Yang H, Fang Z, Wei Y, Hu Y, Calin GA, Kantarjian HM, et al. Levels of miR-29b do not predict for response in patients with acute myelogenous leukemia treated with the combination of 5-azacytidine, valproic acid, and ATRA. American Journal of Hematology. 2011;**86**:237-238. DOI: 10.1002/ajh.21937

[47] Butrym A, Rybka J, Baczyńska D, Poręba R, Mazur G, Kuliczkowski K. Expression of microRNA-181 determines response to treatment with azacitidine and predicts survival in elderly patients with acute myeloid leukaemia. Oncology Letters. 2016;**12**: 2296-2300. DOI: 10.3892/ol.2016.4970

[48] Kim Y, Cheong JW, Kim YK, Eom JI, Jeung HK, Kim SJ, et al. Serum microRNA-21 as a potential biomarker for response to hypomethylating agents in myelodysplastic syndromes. PLoS One. 2014;**9**:e86933. DOI: 10.1371/journal.pone.0086933

[49] Liu H, Pattie P, Chandrasekara S, Spencer A, Dear AE. Epigenetic regulation of miRNA-124 and multiple downstream targets is associated with treatment response in myeloid malignancies. Oncology Letters. 2016; **12**(3):2175-2180. DOI: 10.3892/ol.2016.4912

[50] Wang H, Zhang TT, Jin S, Liu H, Zhang X, Ruan CG, et al. Pyrosequencing quantified methylation level of miR-124 predicts shorter survival for patients with myelodysplastic syndrome. Clinical Epigenetics. 2017;**9**:91. DOI: 10.1186/s13148-017-0388-5

[51] Krejcik Z, Belickova M, Hrustincova A, Votavova H, Jonasova A, Cermak J, et al. MicroRNA profiles as predictive markers of response to azacitidine therapy in myelodysplastic syndromes and acute myeloid leukemia. Cancer Biomarkers. 2018;**22**:101-110. DOI: 10.3233/CBM-171029

[52] Zuo Z, Calin GA, de Paula HM, Medeiros LJ, Fernandez MH, Shimizu M, et al. Circulating microRNAs let-7a and miR-16 predict progression-free survival and overall survival in patients with myelodysplastic syndrome. Blood. 2011;**118**:413-415. DOI: 10.1182/blood-2011-01-330704

[53] Zuo Z, Maiti S, Hu S, Loghavi S, Calin GA, Garcia-Manero G, et al. Plasma circulating-microRNA profiles are useful for assessing prognosis in patients with cytogenetically normal myelodysplastic syndromes. Modern Pathology. 2015;**28**:373-382. DOI: 10.1038/modpathol.2014.108

[54] Dostalova Merkerova M, Hrustincova A, Krejcik Z, Votavova H, Ratajova E, Cermak J, et al. Microarray

profiling defines circulating microRNAs associated with myelodysplastic syndromes. Neoplasma. 2017;**64**:571-578. DOI: 10.4149/neo_2017_411

[55] Shi X, Sun M, Liu H, Yao Y, Song Y. Long non-coding RNAs: A new frontier in the study of human diseases. Cancer Letters. 2013;**339**:159-166. DOI: 10.1016/j.canlet.2013.06.013

[56] Volders PJ, Verheggen K, Menschaert G, Vandepoele K, Martens L, Vandesompele J, et al. An update on LNCipedia: A database for annotated human lncRNA sequences. Nucleic Acids Research. 2015;**43**:4363-4364. DOI: 10.1093/nar/gkv295

[57] Quek XC, Thomson DW, Maag JL, Bartonicek N, Signal B, Clark MB, et al. lncRNAdb v2.0: Expanding the reference database for functional long noncoding RNAs. Nucleic Acids Research. 2015;**43**:168-173. DOI: 10.1093/nar/gku988

[58] Dinger ME, Pang KC, Mercer TR, Crowe ML, Grimmond SM, Mattick JS. NRED: A database of long noncoding RNA expression. Nucleic Acids Research. 2009;**37**:122-126. DOI: 10.1093/nar/gkn617

[59] Wagner LA, Christensen CJ, Dunn DM, Spangrude GJ, Georgelas A, Kelley L, et al. EGO, a novel, noncoding RNA gene, regulates eosinophil granule protein transcript expression. Blood. 2007;**109**:5191-5198. DOI: 10.1182/blood-2006-06-027987

[60] Brannan CI, Dees EC, Ingram RS, Tilghman SM. The product of the H19 gene may function as an RNA. Molecular and Cellular Biology. 1990;**10**:28-36

[61] Venkatraman A, He XC, Thorvaldsen JL, Sugimura R, Perry JM, Tao F, et al. Maternal imprinting at the H19-Igf2 locus maintains adult haematopoietic stem cell quiescence. Nature. 2013;**500**:345-349. DOI: 10.1038/nature12303

[62] Zhang X, Lian Z, Padden C, Gerstein MB, Rozowsky J, Snyder M, et al. A myelopoiesis-associated regulatory intergenic noncoding RNA transcript within the human HOXA cluster. Blood. 2009;**113**:2526-2534. DOI: 10.1182/blood-2008-06-162164

[63] Hu W, Yuan B, Flygare J, Lodish HF. Long noncoding RNA-mediated anti-apoptotic activity in murine erythroid terminal differentiation. Genes & Development. 2011;**25**:2573-2578. DOI: 10.1101/gad.178780.111

[64] Gomez JA, Wapinski OL, Yang YW, Bureau JF, Gopinath S, Monack DM, et al. The NeST long ncRNA controls microbial susceptibility and epigenetic activation of the interferon-gamma locus. Cell. 2013;**152**:743-754. DOI: 10.1016/j.cell.2013.01.015

[65] Carpenter S, Aiello D, Atianand MK, Ricci EP, Gandhi P, Hall LL, et al. A long noncoding RNA mediates both activation and repression of immune response genes. Science. 2013;**341**:789-792. DOI: 10.1126/science.1240925

[66] Zhang L, Xu HG, Lu C. A novel long non-coding RNA T-ALL-R-LncR1 knockdown and Par-4 cooperate to induce cellular apoptosis in T-cell acute lymphoblastic leukemia cells. Leukemia & Lymphoma. 2014;**55**:1373-1382. DOI: 10.3109/10428194.2013.829574

[67] Trimarchi T, Bilal E, Ntziachristos P, Fabbri G, Dalla-Favera R, Tsirigos A, et al. Genome-wide mapping and characterization of Notch-regulated long noncoding RNAs in acute leukemia. Cell. 2014;**158**:593-606. DOI: 10.1016/j.cell.2014.05.049

[68] Gupta RA, Shah N, Wang KC, Kim J, Horlings HM, Wong DJ, et al. Long non-coding RNA HOTAIR reprograms chromatin state to promote cancer

metastasis. Nature. 2010;**464**:1071-1076. DOI: 10.1038/nature08975

[69] Zhu L, Liu J, Ma S, Zhang S. Long noncoding RNA MALAT-1 can predict metastasis and a poor prognosis: A meta-analysis. Pathology Oncology Research. 2015;**21**:1259-1264. DOI: 10.1007/s12253-015-9960-5

[70] Benetatos L, Hatzimichael E, Dasoula A, Dranitsaris G, Tsiara S, Syrrou M, et al. CpG methylation analysis of the MEG3 and SNRPN imprinted genes in acute myeloid leukemia and myelodysplastic syndromes. Leukemia Research. 2010; **34**:148-153. DOI: 10.1016/j.leukres.2009.06.019

[71] Zhang Z, Liu T, Wang K, Qu X, Pang Z, Liu S, et al. Down-regulation of long non-coding RNA MEG3 indicates an unfavorable prognosis in non-small cell lung cancer: Evidence from the GEO database. Gene. 2017;**630**:49-58. DOI: 10.1016/j.gene.2017.08.001

[72] Tian ZZ, Guo XJ, Zhao YM, Fang Y. Decreased expression of long non-coding RNA MEG3 acts as a potential predictor biomarker in progression and poor prognosis of osteosarcoma. International Journal of Clinical and Experimental Pathology. 2015;**8**:15138-15142

[73] Yildirim E, Kirby JE, Brown DE, Mercier FE, Sadreyev RI, Scadden DT, et al. Xist RNA is a potent suppressor of hematologic cancer in mice. Cell. 2013; **152**:727-742. DOI: 10.1016/j.cell.2013.01.034

[74] Liu K, Beck D, Thoms JAI, Liu L, Zhao W, Pimanda JE, et al. Annotating function to differentially expressed LincRNAs in myelodysplastic syndrome using a network-based method. Bioinformatics. 2017;**33**:2622-2630. DOI: 10.1093/bioinformatics/btx280

[75] Yao CY, Chen CH, Huang HH, Hou HA, Lin CC, Tseng MH, et al. A 4-lncRNA scoring system for prognostication of adult myelodysplastic syndromes. Blood Advances. 2017;**1**:1505-1516. DOI: 10.1182/bloodadvances.2017008284

[76] Beck D, Ayers S, Wen J, Brandl MB, Pham TD, Webb P, et al. Integrative analysis of next generation sequencing for small non-coding RNAs and transcriptional regulation in myelodysplastic syndromes. BMC Medical Genomics. 2011;**4**:19. DOI: 10.1186/1755-8794-4-19

[77] Klattenhoff C, Theurkauf W. Biogenesis and germline functions of piRNAs. Development. 2008;**135**:3-9. DOI: 10.1242/dev.006486

[78] Pavon-Eternod M, Gomes S, Geslain R, Dai Q, Rosner MR, Pan T. tRNA over-expression in breast cancer and functional consequences. Nucleic Acids Research. 2009;**37**:7268-7280. DOI: 10.1093/nar/gkp787

[79] van Raam BJ, Salvesen GS. Transferring death: A role for tRNA in apoptosis regulation. Molecular Cell. 2010;**37**:591-592. DOI: 10.1016/j.molcel.2010.02.001

[80] Guo Y, Bosompem A, Mohan S, Erdogan B, Ye F, Vickers KC, et al. Transfer RNA detection by small RNA deep sequencing and disease association with myelodysplastic syndromes. BMC Genomics. 2015;**16**:727. DOI: 10.1186/s12864-015-1929-y

[81] Shah MY, Ferrajoli A, Sood AK, Lopez-Berestein G, Calin GA. microRNA therapeutics in cancer—An emerging concept. eBioMedicine. 2016;

12:34-42. DOI: 10.1016/j.ebiom.2016.09.017

[82] Bader AG. miR-34—A microRNA replacement therapy is headed to the clinic. Frontiers in Genetics. 2012;**3**:120. DOI: 10.3389/fgene.2012.00120

[83] Foss FM, Querfeld C, Porcu P, Kim YH, Pacheco T, Halwani AS. Phase 1 trial evaluating MRG-106, a synthetic inhibitor of microRNA-155, in patients with cutaneous t-cell lymphoma (CTCL). Journal of Clinical Oncology. 2017;**35**(15_suppl):7564-7564. DOI: 10.1200/JCO.2017.35.15_suppl.7564